I'm Not Crazy, I'm Just a Little Unwell

My Journey Through Chronic Fatigue Syndrome

Leigh Hatcher

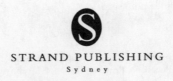

STRAND PUBLISHING

Sydney

I'm Not Crazy, I'm Just a Little Unwell
Copyright © 2005 by Leigh Hatcher

First published by Strand Publishing 2005

ISBN: 1876825359

Distributed in Australia by:
Family Reading Publications
B100 Ring Road
Ballarat Victoria 3352
Phone: 03 5334 3244
Fax: 03 5334 3299
Email: orders@familyreading.com.au

Most Bible quotations are taken from *The Holy Bible, New International Version®*, Copyright © 1973, 1978, 1984 by the International Bible Society. Used by permission of Zondervan Publishing House. Job 14:7 and 2 Timothy 1:7 are taken from *The Holy Bible, New King James Version*, Copyright © 1982 by Thomas Nelson, Inc. Used by permission. All rights reserved.

Excerpts in chapter 9 are from *Surviving Survival* by M. Little, C. Jordens, K. Paul & E. Sayers, Choice Books, Marrickville 2001. Used by permission.

Quote from 'Unwell' by Rob Thomas, © 2002 Bidnis Inc. For Australia and New Zealand: EMI Music Publishing Australia Pty Ltd (ABN 83 000 040 951), PO Box 481, Spit Junction NSW 2008. International copyright secured. All rights reserved. Used by permission.

Photographs:
Cover photograph by David Oliver Photography. Used by permission.
The sacking of Gough Whitlam, courtesy of *The Canberra Times*. Used by permission.
Leigh Hatcher with Channel Seven news crew, courtesy of the Seven Network. Used by permission.
Leigh Hatcher at the Cole Classic, John Doughty—Hot Shots Photography. Used by permission.

Edited by Owen Salter
Cover design by Joy Lankshear
Typesetting by Midland Typesetters, Maryborough, Victoria
Printed in Australia by McPherson's Printing Group, Maryborough, Victoria

'I'm not crazy, I'm just a little unwell'
Rob Thomas—'Unwell'
Matchbox Twenty

To Amy

With thanks to my best friend, Meredith, and to Tristan, Amy, Johanna and Sophie. Special thanks also to Jill and Ian, Fiona, Pauline, Maurice, Penny and Peter, Harry, Helen, Lyn, Ken and Patsy, Mark and Susan, Drs Gary Franks, John D'Arcy and Robert Loblay and my fabulous editor, Owen Salter.

Contents

Preface

Many thousands, perhaps millions, around the world suffer silently with chronic fatigue syndrome. They suffer terribly from the illness itself—there is much physical pain. They also suffer great loss, forced to endure shattered hopes, plans and relationships.

Most of the time, though, they will tell you that the worst suffering, beyond all the physical hurt, comes from widespread misunderstanding of the illness and from the suspicion people have about its reality and therefore about the validity of the sufferer.

Those of us with chronic fatigue syndrome—or CFS as it is often known—hate the fact that it's 'just' a syndrome. Too often it is written off as being 'all in the mind' or 'just being tired'. Sometimes it's even judged to be a kind of lifestyle choice. If only it were that simple! CFS sufferers try to find other names for the illness, other categories, but in the end it remains 'just' a syndrome. Yet so is SIDS (Sudden Infant Death Syndrome), and so is SARS (Severe Acute Respiratory Syndrome). No one misunderstands either the tangible reality and validity of those syndromes or their devastating consequences.

In the end, CFS sufferers can seldom win out over all the misunderstandings and misguided judgments. They are forced into retreat and often into deep hurt. They are just too ill to keep beating their heads against a brick wall. They are driven into silence, resentment, anger and sometimes depression.

All of this drives my passionate hope for this book—that in some small way it can give CFS sufferers both a voice and validity. I want to show them that they are not alone in their struggles. If my story is able to contribute anything, I hope it can be a voice of acceptance and comfort—a voice of someone who knows the reality of this illness and can communicate that reality on behalf of those whose own voices have been crushed or humiliated into silence by too many suspicions and misjudgments.

I also want to provide CFS sufferers with a resource they can pass on to doubting or puzzled family, friends, neighbours and work colleagues. All these people need to know that the suffering of CFS is more than enough on its own without other people's unsympathetic scepticism. This book is a voice urging acceptance and love, probably over the long haul. It is a voice that rages against the simplistic notion that CFS is 'all in the mind', a cop-out from life or, worst of all, a fraud.

I have two primary desires for the book. First, I want it to be of help to anyone battling CFS—or indeed, any kind of serious, long-term illness or upheaval. I confess to being a pragmatist. My aim is to provide practical insights through real-life experiences that can help make the long haul bearable.

For family and friends of those doing it tough, I offer practical suggestions, often born out of much pain and hurt, about how they can best be alongside those who suffer.

Second, I want to point to the fact that though CFS has been truly a 'wilderness experience' for me, it has never been totally dark— never without hope. Primarily, this hope has come from the way I have been resourced, encouraged and uplifted by an unshakeable faith in God. This part of my experience will not be shared by everyone who has CFS, but for me it is simply impossible to leave it out and still write a true account of all I have been through.

My journey through CFS raises honest questions, not only about why we suffer, but also about how there can be help and hope, even meaning, in the darkest days. It is a reporter's story written in the style I know best, a factual narrative based on 500,000 words of diaries I recorded through my illness. I hope you find it an honest, accessible and authentic read.

Of course, no two CFS stories will ever be the same. I don't imagine that my story or my way out of this illness is typical. There is no typical story. However, the syndrome is very real—and if my story can affirm, empower and encourage other sufferers, it will be worth the battles I have been through with this terrible illness.

Leigh Hatcher

CHAPTER 1

Into the Wilderness

Monday, 19 January 1998, 3.00 p.m.

I can pinpoint the exact instant my life turned upside down. I was in the middle of a two-week holiday at one of the golden beaches that line the east coast of Australia. I have been to lots of impressive places around the world, but for me few can match the simple beauty and serenity of MacMasters Beach on the central coast of New South Wales. We were staying with my mother, who had retired there with my late father in the early '90s.

I am a man of simple needs when it comes to a holiday—surf, sun, sleep and good food. My daily routine on our beach holidays went like this: up at 6.00 a.m. for fifty laps of the tidal pool, back to the house for breakfast, back down to the beach with the family for the morning, lunch, a ten-minute nap, back to the beach for the afternoon, then dinner and more sleep. Bliss!

On this particular day, though, I woke from my ten-minute nap two hours later, feeling as if I'd been run over by a truck. I felt all the aches of a typical flu.

We pressed on with the rest of the day. That night we drove to Sydney for a friend's sixtieth birthday party and then returned to the coast. For the rest of that week I felt below par, slightly smashed though not ill enough to immediately rush off to the doctor. I remember starkly feeling a strong and sudden reluctance to press on with my laps of the pool or take the plunge into the clear, sparkling surf. For years I had had a love affair with lap swimming and the surf, but now the thought of any extra exertion—and especially of the cold water—seemed more than my body could handle.

I have since become convinced that your body tells you what it needs. My body was going into self-preservation mode.

We returned home from our holiday at the end of the week with me still feeling below par. It did not seem that serious, but I was clearly not well. I was surprisingly tired, achy and slightly nauseous. Facing a long weekend when medical help would be hard to get, I thought it best to see the doctor. He sent me off for some routine blood tests, saying it was probably a virus which time would simply heal.

The next morning I took a couple of our kids to a Sydney beach, though again I did not feel able to take the plunge into the surf. As I sat on the sand, my mobile phone went off. It was my doctor, rather alarmed. He said one of the blood tests had shown abnormal liver function levels and concluded that I must have come down with hepatitis. I was to rest and be very careful of any close contact with other people, especially kissing. He would order some new tests and I should not go back to work as planned the following Monday.

The further tests showed it was not hepatitis A, B or C. I seemed to have somehow come across a virus that had simply gone to my liver. The doctor ordered me to take two weeks off work and rest.

The fortnight passed quickly. By that time I was becoming a bit agitated to get on with my life again, especially my swimming.

But my body had other plans. I was still not at all well. The flu-like aches and fatigue continued, and there were often times of the day when I would become inexplicably worse. I had lived a highly active life and loved exercise, with fifteen minutes of weight training every morning and swimming up to five kilometres each week. Now suddenly the simplest trip to the shops left me debilitated.

There was nowhere to go but back to bed. The doctor gave me another week off.

At the end of that week, our family went away for the weekend to the beach with six other families from our neighbourhood. Our four kids are Tristan, Amy, Johanna and Sophie. At the time they were sixteen, fourteen, eleven and eight. My wife Meredith and I were in the midst of a busy, demanding yet delightful time with our family. Our neighbourhood was like a big community, so the weekend was to be a great getaway for us all.

By this stage I was beginning to be optimistic that my health was starting to turn the corner. I had been tentatively trying to take on more and more activity and getting away with it—at least some of the time. We drove up on the Friday night, and I thought it was safe enough to start lifting the dietary restrictions I'd been advised to follow. Like everyone else, we stopped for a dinner of takeaway burgers on the way. Next day we had a leisurely morning down at the beach. So far so good.

Then we had a BBQ lunch—and without warning I started feeling very unwell again. Aches and fatigue began to overwhelm me. I went to bed and spent the afternoon in more physical trouble than ever. I slept and then woke with the now-familiar feeling of being run over by a truck. I slept some more and woke again feeling terrible. I spent the rest of the day like that, despairing that I had missed an enjoyable afternoon at the beach. I wasn't much fun that night either, and we ended up returning home the next day more and more frustrated that this 'thing' was not going away.

It was now one month since the original viral illness hit and two weeks since the doctor said I should be able to return to work. I was one of the front line news reporters for the Seven Television Network in Australia, and my enforced absence from my job was a growing frustration. I had been at Channel Seven as a reporter and newsreader for just on ten years and I loved my work. It was challenging, stimulating and varied—rewarding both personally and financially. I was highly regarded, being, among many other things, the Seven Network's Olympic correspondent right from the very early days of Sydney's bid for the 2000 Olympic Games. We were now two-and-a-half years away from the big event. It was all set to be a career highlight.

I had always prided myself on being a committed, resourceful and effective journalist. I would rather spend a day out on the road, facing the many demanding challenges of TV journalism, than sit around all day waiting for the 'big story' to hit and end up doing nothing. So after one month of being ill, I began to get the guilts. My bosses were most understanding, and since they knew my work ethic well, there was no pressure to return until I was fully well again.

I deeply appreciated their support and care, yet I became more and more agitated that I couldn't shake this 'thing' and jump back on the bandwagon of life and work.

Over the next week or so I went back to my GP a couple of times. I reported to him the symptoms I was continuing to suffer. There were aches all over my body like a bad dose of the flu (though it was clearly not the flu). Accompanying the aches were what I described as large 'crashes' at various parts of the day. They were like blood sugar crashes, as if I had done a hard day's work on little food then had to do another eight hours before eating again. When these crashes hit, there was nowhere for me to be except in bed. I was unable to pinpoint why they happened or predict when they would strike.

I noted other bewildering things about my body. One was how awful I felt when I woke in the morning. I had always been a morning person, bounding out of bed at 5.30 or 6.00 a.m., frequently down to the pool for a two-kilometre swim. Now, most mornings I woke up feeling as if an elephant was sitting on me.

I also found that for most of the day I was growlingly hungry. This was a marked and consistent difference in the way my body had always operated. Yet although I was exercising less and eating more, I was quite dramatically losing weight. I'd always had to work hard to keep my weight down; now it was falling off.

In addition, for some reason I was really struggling to handle stressful situations as well as I used to. It was only the usual argy-bargy of family life. But after a career of facing down impossibly stressful, sometimes life-threatening situations, I would blow up at my family as never before.

All of this I faithfully reported to my increasingly puzzled doctor. I explained that despite these baffling and draining symptoms, each morning I determinedly got out of bed, went for a walk (more like a shuffle) around the block, and tried to get on with the day. He sent me off for new tests.

They all came back 'normal', but normal was the last thing I was feeling.

Unable to take it any further, my GP referred me to a liver specialist, who ordered still more tests. They too came back normal. He ended up labelling me 'mystery man' and became clearly frustrated with my lack of progress. In one phone call he expressed a surprising level of agitation. 'Well, I've done everything I can for you and have sent you off for every test I can think of,' he said. 'The only other test I could order is an AIDS test.'

I felt sharply accused of being less than frank with him, to the extent I could be hiding AIDS. I was shocked at his accusatory tone, as if it were up to me to get better myself.

By now I had been off work for two months. I had never experienced anything like this. I continued to feel acutely guilty, though still my news director extended to me the most generous and gracious consideration. Fortunately, a good and long-standing friend, Dr John D'Arcy, a general practitioner and the medical reporter on our news team, began to visit me at home. He could clearly see how ill I was and urged me only to return to work when I could.

Notwithstanding all this, I decided that my best way forward was to see if I could push my body back into real life again. Perhaps it needed a kick-start. After eight weeks away I negotiated a partial return to the newsroom on half days.

It was great to be back among colleagues and good to be seen on the television again, though I still looked pretty ill. Initially I was frustrated that more often than not I was assigned to be 'on the bench', waiting for the big story that frequently did not eventuate. I felt they were being too protective. I'm sure our medical reporter had a lot to do with that.

My wife's birthday, 10 April, raised new alarm bells. We had her family over to lunch and didn't eat until 2.00 p.m. As we waited and waited, I started to spiral into one of my crashes. But it was unlike any I had experienced before. Accompanying the crash was a mounting rage about the lateness of lunch. This was all too much and something entirely outside my experience and control.

When I finally gobbled down the meal, the spiral continued. I had to excuse myself and head to bed, where I wasted the rest of the afternoon in a great deal of physical trouble. My whole body felt toxic. Each time I woke I seemed to emerge into a half-conscious daze only to sink back into sleep again. Sadly for Meredith, it was not a very happy birthday.

After attempting a number of half days at work, I decided to try a full day. It was an enjoyable shoot at a lakeside resort for a leisure and lifestyle show put together by the newsroom. Blessedly, I had a producer working with me organising all the logistics and components of the story, because for much of the shoot I lay in the car feeling like I was dying. Such pain all over my body. I would sleep, do an interview, sleep some more, do some on-camera work and then go back for more sleep.

This was an all-too-familiar scenario from my days at home, but now I was frustrated and angry that it was on show before my work colleagues. It seemed as if my time-honoured work ethic had been completely overrun by this lingering illness that kept on throwing up 'normal' test results. I returned home that day physically devastated, and yet again went straight to bed.

Part of my daily routine for nearly a decade had been a brisk walk to work. We lived just two kilometres from Channel Seven Sydney. The day after our leisure shoot, I decided to resume my walks to work. I was fiercely determined that this 'thing' would not get the better of me.

Again I woke feeling awful but pressed on to work regardless. I lasted one hour. Once again I felt that dreadful toxic feeling, as if something poisonous was running through my blood stream. I thought I had become good at hiding it but it must have been evident in my physical appearance. The news director took one look at me and ordered me into a camera crew car to be taken straight home.

At last I was forced to run up the white flag and accept that still, some three months after contracting my original virus, I was not well. Despite the best will in the world, I kept on crashing, so debilitated. And I had no idea why.

Neither did I know that all this was just the beginning, and that stretching out in front of me was the hardest journey I had ever had to undertake. In fact, I had entered a wilderness. It would be a long time before I would be able to emerge again.

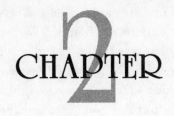

CHAPTER 2

In the Fast Lane

Monday, 12 November 1973, 11.30 a.m.

My love affair with journalism began one morning late in 1973 when I stepped into the newsroom at radio station 2GB.

The previous Friday I had finished the last of my Higher School Certificate exams. I'd had a pretty underwhelming school education due to an overwhelming lack of interest. Six months before the final exams, my despairing parents booked me an appointment with the school counsellor to frighten me into doing at least some study. He warned that unless I put in a minimum of four hours' work every night, I would be a failure in the exams and in life generally. This dire prediction had no practical effect, and the only real study I ended up doing was in the final two weeks. I was a good crammer.

Only one thing stirred me: the stage. Whether it was musicals or dramas, chorus parts or lead roles, I was there, revelling in it all. The fun, the music, the camaraderie, the mounting tension of approaching opening night, the smell of the make-up—it all captivated and consumed me. Whenever anyone asked me what I wanted to do after high school, I would say, 'Show business'.

My parents wisely guided me to consider radio or television rather than the vagaries of the acting world. I went for a number of interviews and ended up being able to choose between office boy jobs at two Sydney radio stations, 2GB and 2UW. At the time, 2GB was the headquarters of what was then a considerable force in Australian radio, the Macquarie Radio Network. My parents' advice was to go with the strength of such a large and well-established national organisation, and so it was that this young, green school leaver turned up for work on Monday, 12 November 1973.

My duties were relatively simple. I was one of four office boys whose job was to deliver documents and run errands around the 2GB building and through the city of Sydney. At the same time, I'd be getting to know the various roles and departments within the radio station so I could get an idea of what career I might want to follow.

It didn't take me long to find out. The instant I stepped into the newsroom late that first morning, I was captivated. I stood there with a silly grin on my face and a sense of wonder. There was lots of noise—the clatter of clunky old typewriters, tapes being spooled, feeds being recorded, phones jangling. One entire room was consumed with the relentless march of telex tape being fed through up to ten machines, sending out the latest news to radio stations across the country. There was also lots of shouting as these increasingly frantic and focused people approached one of the highlights of the day, the midday bulletin. I could feel the tension.

In one frozen moment in time I was intoxicated. It was a kind of love at first sight.

In my ill-defined desire to get into 'show business', journalism had never made it onto my radar. It was an entirely different business in the early '70s from what it would become in future years. Journalists were mostly older men, grumpy, hard living and certainly hard drinking. I only knew one woman journalist. The job of a journalist had no particular 'profile', and there were none of the stellar salaries that people in the business would later be able to command.

Suddenly there could not have been a greater contrast between my lack of work and focus at school and the iron determination I now had to join the newsroom. I grabbed every opportunity to do the newsroom deliveries and hung around there like the proverbial bad smell. I asked anyone I could how to go about gaining a cadetship.

Pretty soon the difference between the excitement of the newsroom and the grinding ordinariness of being an office boy started to tell. There was a clear pecking order among the office boys, based purely on longevity in the job. When you made it to 'executive' office boy, almost your entire time was spent running personal errands for the two women in charge of the office boys and for their cronies. By then you knew exactly which biscuits to buy at the David Jones food hall and especially the right sort of gravy beef to buy for their pets. No doubt it was character building, but it drove me crazy. I could not wait to get free.

My break finally came. After much pleading and nagging, the news director awarded me a cadetship. I'm sure I got the job to shut me up and get me out of his hair as much as anything else. At the end of my first day in the newsroom, I walked to the train station with the newsroom's editor. I asked him if he had one piece of advice on such a day. His response was instantaneous: 'Never panic.' Although it didn't mean much to me at the time, this turned out to be the best piece of wisdom for surviving in a crazy, over-stressed business.

I took to the job of being a journalist like a shark to mullet, working all sorts of crazy hours, seven days a week. Soon I was out on the road reporting, and then came one of the most terrifying of moments—my first 'voice report'. I was actually on the radio! I rang my parents, who were in an almost perpetual state of astonishment at the total turnaround in my work ethic. I was now doing something I loved.

Mid-1974 was a very important time in the business of journalism. Richard Nixon was in terminal decline as the President of the United States, relentlessly being brought undone by a new creature, the 'investigative journalist'.

As I caught the train to work each day, I would devour all the intricacies of the Watergate scandal from my father's copies of *Time Magazine*. It was intoxicating to consider that I was being trained in a profession that was demonstrating such potent power in bringing down the US President. I remember standing in the newsroom awestruck by a moment in history, listening as we put to air Richard Nixon's resignation speech on 8 August 1974.

On reflection, I consider Watergate to be one of journalism's great turning points. Through it, journalists gained a notoriety, power and profile that rapidly transformed the profession. Soon it became one of the hottest jobs, with salaries to match. Seemingly endless opportunities and outlets opened up for reporters, especially in the electronic media. Within a few years, journalists were also brought into the inner circle of governments to try to beat the media at its own game.

It all ended up having a profound effect on how societies and nations operate. It was truly a gift to be part of this exciting new world.

Around this time, I had one delightful and consuming distraction from my busy work life. I resumed an on-again, off-again romance with Meredith Bridgford, who had been a constant for much of my childhood. We were in the same kindergarten class at school, and our parents both had holiday houses at MacMasters Beach, where we would sometimes indulge in a brief summer romance. We also went to the same Sunday school and ultimately youth fellowship at a local church.

Our new romance stuck this time—it was so right. Already knowing each other so well, our love for each other deepened quickly. It was mushy yet solid, and within a couple of months we were talking about options for when we could marry. We decided to wait for three years until she finished her science degree and became a physiotherapist.

All our plans were soon tested, though, by a simple phone call from my news director offering me the job of chief political correspondent for the Macquarie Radio Network in Australia's capital city, Canberra. I was so stunned after I hung up the phone that I lay on the floor giggling and gibbering in disbelief. I was all of nineteen years old and barely knew anything of politics. I had never even contemplated moving away from home. It was preposterous—yet how could I say no?

I had already learnt the first imperative of journalism—you sink or you swim. So far I had been swimming, though sometimes with only my head above water. What lay ahead was an experience of being thrown in the deep end that was more scary than almost anything else I've come across in this frequently very scary business.

Meredith and I had to work out quickly whether this would be the end of our new and deeply committed attachment to each other. Neither of us could contemplate walking away from the relationship, so I committed myself to the five-hour drive between Canberra and Sydney each weekend to see her (and to have my mum wash my clothes!). I cried when I left home—mainly as I farewelled my trusty dog, Deane.

Arriving in Canberra in August 1975 I walked headlong into my baptism of fire. Gough Whitlam had been Australia's Prime Minister for nearly three years and was in the same sort of terminal decline as Richard Nixon exactly one year before. In Whitlam's case it was more political incompetence and manufactured scandal than the criminality and cover up of Watergate. Once again journalists, fired by the intoxicating power that had brought down an American President, were in the forefront of reporting and sometimes initiating Whitlam's decline.

My first day at work in Parliament House was budget day 1975. Eventually the Opposition parties blocked that budget in the Senate, effectively denying the Whitlam Government the money it needed to run the country. After three solid months of 'constitutional crisis', and much to the amazement of most people, the Governor-General, Sir John Kerr, sacked the Prime Minister. It was arguably the greatest upheaval in Australia's political history and I was caught in the middle of it, having to make sense of it all for a national radio audience. By this time I was all of twenty!

On the day Whitlam was sacked, 11 November 1975, an angry crowd of hundreds was spontaneously drawn to the front steps of Parliament House after they heard the big news. The Governor-General's official secretary, David Smith, appeared to read the proclamation dissolving the parliament and calling a national election. His short speech was swamped by boos and abuse. Then suddenly the imposing figure of Gough Whitlam strode out and stood behind the hapless David Smith. The crowd went berserk.

That one chaotic moment was captured in a now-renowned black and white photograph. It would become the defining image of that historic event—and there next to Gough and David Smith is this bearded and slightly ruffled twenty-year-old radio reporter. That photo has become my one great claim to fame. With each new decade of that day since 1975, I have been rung by radio stations and other journalists to be interviewed about what it was like to be there. The image has made it onto coffee cups, tea towels and even into my kids' school history textbooks—much to their serious embarrassment.

The events of that year put me onto the fast track of an already accelerating career. People would often ask me where I wanted to end up in journalism, and I would say that one day I would like to be a 'news executive'. This happened much earlier than I expected. At twenty-one I became news editor of Radio 2CA, the Macquarie Network station in Canberra.

Meredith and I fulfilled our dreams of three years before when we married at the end of 1977. Within a year we moved to Adelaide where I became the news director of the Macquarie Network station there, 5DN. As it was one of the pioneering 'news-talk' stations, management felt it was logical to put a journalist in charge of the station's programming. Within eighteen months of my arrival at 5DN, I was appointed director of programs and news.

Television first made it onto my radar in 1981, when I was offered the job of political correspondent for the Seven Network, again in Canberra. It was a very tough decision to leave radio, my first professional love. But I was becoming more and more disillusioned with the life of an executive. It seemed to be a never-ending round of meetings and kicking people in the backside. In my mid-twenties I was still young enough to step back easily into the job I knew and did best—reporting.

Within months of our move back to Canberra, our first child, Tristan, was born safely into the world.

Television was a whole new and intimidating world. But it offered rich rewards and great professional fulfilment, including numbers of overseas trips with prime ministers and foreign ministers. After two years in Canberra I was offered the job of European Correspondent for the Seven Network. With Meredith three months pregnant with our second child, Amy, we packed up to move to London on a two-year contract. The fast track gathered speed at every new turn. War, bombings, riots, political upheavals and lots of delightful colour stories became my almost total preoccupation throughout Eastern and Western Europe between 1983 and 1985.

The job of a foreign correspondent is as exhausting as it is intoxicating, however, and the end of my contract in London enabled me to seriously consider a more balanced life. I negotiated a return to radio with 5DN in Adelaide. At first I went back to be part of their newsroom, and soon after I became one half of a news-talk breakfast radio program. Ultimately I became the sole host. Our third child, Johanna, was born in 1987.

Within a couple of years the Australian media began to go through a number of great upheavals, mainly because of corporate takeovers and some corporate disasters. As networking gobbled up more and more jobs and outlets, it became clear to me that the writing was on the wall for interesting opportunities in cities like Adelaide. After a change of management and philosophy at 5DN, I called a friend in Sydney to explore options about returning to the Seven Network. They welcomed me with open arms like a prodigal son returning to the family fold.

After fourteen years away from Sydney the time was right for a return to be closer to our families. Sophie, our third daughter and fourth child, was born there in 1990.

I began work in the Sydney newsroom as a senior reporter and soon took on the initially terrifying job of reading the news on weekends. Each day at work had its fill of death, doom and destruction, the usual fare for a commercial television news service. I was also appointed the Seven Network's chief Olympic reporter. It was a prized position as Seven had already established itself as 'The Olympic Network', having secured the broadcast rights to the Year 2000 Games, for which Sydney had launched a major bid.

After much lobbying by Sydney and a number of overseas trips for me, we found ourselves in Monte Carlo in September 1993, where the prize of hosting the Year 2000 Games was to be awarded. We spent twelve days reporting on every twist and turn of the Olympic bid roller coaster. Most people were expecting the overwhelming force of Beijing's bid to triumph. Yet when we gathered at the Monte Carlo convention hall for the big announcement, the diminutive IOC President, Juan Antonio Samaranch, uttered those now immortal words: 'And de winner is Syderney.' I was in shock and tears. Suddenly I had to completely re-write the story I had already sketched out in my mind, expecting Beijing to win.

It was a truly exhilarating time. What a prize for Sydney! It was a heady experience reporting it all back to a city that was going ballistic. For the next three days we ran on adrenalin and a total of about three hours sleep, arriving back in Australia entirely exhausted but elated.

I had now spent twenty years on the front line of broadcast media reporting around the world. There were a few great triumphs like Monte Carlo, but for the most part there were great tragedies. My stories often dealt with people who were living an ordinary, every-day existence until suddenly their lives were turned upside down. All through, I had simply been the reporter and never imagined my charmed life to be in any way challenged.

All this changed late one afternoon in the Blue Mountains west of Sydney.

Saturday, 8 January 1994 was a day of soaring temperatures, crashing humidity and strong blustery winds. For more than a week Sydney had been in the grip of its worst bushfire crisis for decades.

Early in the day, the Channel Seven helicopter flew a camera crew and me to the Blue Mountains. It was an ominously quiet trip as we contemplated what lay ahead of us. Our chopper was buffeted by wind gusts, a sure sign that all the dire forecasts for the day were already being fulfilled. An enormous fire front was marching relent-lessly down one of the largest valleys in the mountains, and all the experts were predicting a horror day.

For much of the day we sat and waited with mounting frustration as the deadline for our main evening news approached. So far the fire front had been burning in inaccessible bush, fortunately sparing a number of mountain communities.

Around 4.30 p.m. everything changed. There was a sudden and

urgent mobilisation of the fire crews around us. As they rushed off with sirens blaring, we followed closely behind. They positioned themselves facing a high two-kilometre long ridge. Within minutes an unbelievable and awesome sight met our eyes. Along its entire length, the top of the ridge exploded into flames. Towering gum trees seventy metres tall erupted, the flames leaping another seventy metres into the air. Then they started heading straight down the valley.

Quickly I did what we call a 'piece to camera', a couple of lines of me talking to the camera, trying to convey the drama of the moment. I did several takes as the flames raced nearer.

Abruptly a number of fire crews were called away to an area under even greater threat. We sent our tape off to a nearby 'link truck' that was beaming material back to the Sydney newsroom, then turned to follow the fire crews—and walked into hell.

The fire front was now consuming bush at the rear of a whole street of houses. Some of the houses were already ablaze. We had to use the high beams of our headlights to find our way through the smoke. The cameraman, soundman and I leapt out of the car and ran into the thick of it. The noise was like nothing I had ever experienced. The flames, fired by a fearsome wind, gave off a roar something like a steam train under full power—unstoppable, unrelenting and absolutely terrifying. Visibility in some areas was reduced to only a couple of metres.

Within minutes I had become separated from the camera crew. Alone in the searing heat, I thought I was about to die. I faced a terrible choice: to run for my life or to try to link back up with the crew. I chose to run and run, though starved of oxygen by the all-consuming wall of smoke. At one stage I wondered if I was going to choke to death, as many do in serious fires.

I emerged into a precious area of clearer air and collected my breath and my thoughts. I had no idea what had happened to the crew and felt the responsibility to try to find them. I ran back into the chaos, screaming out their names. Amid all the noise and confusion I eventually heard them yelling back at me. I felt such relief.

Still unable to see much, we followed the sounds of each other's screams until we linked back up. I yelled four words, 'We're out of here!', and once again we were running—literally for our lives. As we ran, the cameraman, Scott Lipman, shouted, 'I'm rolling! Do the piece to camera again!' It was the last thing on my mind! But the words of my piece to camera were still fresh in my memory, so I instinctively turned to the camera and blurted them out as we ran, gasping for breath.

Thanks entirely to Lippo's remarkable presence of mind, that piece certainly captured the drama and fear of the moment. It was probably the best fifteen seconds of television I have ever done. It certainly came out of the most terrifying experience I had ever been through as a journalist. I had faced a number of life-threatening situations in the course of my job, but this was by far the worst.

The next day our family took off for another one of our summer holidays at MacMasters Beach. As was often the case, it was a challenging realignment to come down from the adrenalin high of reporting to simply sitting on a beach. But after my near death experience in the Blue Mountains, I felt almost as if I was being given a second chance at life. It made me thoughtful, to say the least.

At the time I was reading a book called *In Pursuit of Excellence*, and I felt acutely the challenge of one particular chapter on goal setting. I had never been much of a goals person, but I thought this could be a useful 'fresh start' to my life. As I contemplated what goals I could set for the years ahead, I thought a good starting point would be the way my life was unfolding in regards to my Christian faith.

I had first embraced Christianity in my mid-teens when my grandfather and a close family friend died within a relatively short time of each other. The only place where I ever heard the issue of death dealt with at all, and dealt with coherently and honestly, was within the context of the Christian faith. There, it was also balanced with hope—hope that death was not the end for those who were connected to God. It seemed a realistic and credible hope, founded on the reality of God, the beauty and design of his world, and his intervention in human history in the person of Jesus Christ.

As an adult I'd found that people were sometimes amused at the apparent contradiction in the term 'Christian journalist', yet I had never felt it necessary to downplay my faith. It gave me a viable reference point both to appreciate the world and to understand myself and those around me. Now, as a result of the profile of my job, I was being increasingly invited to give occasional talks to church groups about how I reconciled my faith with life in the media. I felt highly inadequate for this kind of speaking, so as I sat on the sand staring out to sea, I set myself four goals.

First, I would work on knowing the Bible better. If I was going to speak about it, I would have to understand how it all fitted together and ensure that it shaped my life and character more than I had allowed it to do in the past.

Second, I would learn more about how to put a talk together. I was good at constructing one-minute-ten-second television stories, but preparing a viable and credible twenty-minute talk was a different matter.

Third, I would consider taking a year off full-time work to do some formal theological study. This was the beginning of 1994 and 1997 seemed a good year to aim for. We would have three years to save the money we needed. It would be the year after the 1996 Olympic Games in Atlanta, on which I would be reporting. It would also still be three years out from the Sydney Olympics.

The fourth goal I contemplated dealt with life after the 2000 Olympics. Perhaps I could walk away from full-time work to become something of a free agent, working essentially for myself and leaving time available each week for some kind of itinerant speaking.

All this took just five minutes. There were no flashing lightning bolts, no voices from heaven. I simply got up off the sand and quietly embarked on my four goals with no great fanfare. Only Meredith knew of these plans and warmly embraced them.

Within a few weeks of setting out on these goals, however, I found them being tested. Over the years I've learnt that God works in very tangible yet often amazing ways through the ordinary (and sometimes extraordinary) events of life. And sometimes he pushes those who are his out of their comfort zones as they trust more and more in his all-sufficiency—even though at times it gets pretty scary!

My 'push' came in the form of a call from a politician friend asking me to speak at the annual New South Wales Governor's Prayer Breakfast. This was no little church talk. It was an annual high profile event for 1500 people from the top-end of town among Sydney's political, judicial and corporate life.

The thought of it made me feel like crawling under a rock. Ever since stumbling my way through a high school talk at the age of seventeen, I had been petrified of ever having to get up on my feet again in front of a crowd. Each time I did so it was sheer agony.

Speaking at the Governor's Prayer Breakfast was a million miles away from quick-fire television reporting or performing on stage with a well-rehearsed script. However, if I was serious about pursuing my goals, there seemed little alternative but to accept the invitation. I used a montage of tape from the bushfires, including my brush with death, to illustrate the fleeting nature of life. In the end it went very well.

The next few years continued to go to plan. That one talk at the Governor's Prayer Breakfast opened many doors around New South

Wales and interstate to join the 'speakers' circuit'. Meanwhile, we continued to save and prepare for my year of full-time study.

The Atlanta Olympics came and went, another six weeks of living on adrenalin and very little sleep.

It was my first Olympics, and at the Opening Ceremony I could hardly comprehend the heights of human creativity, performance and organisation on display. It was thrilling, brilliant, breathtaking. The sight of Gladys Knight emerging from under the ground in the very middle of the stadium singing 'Georgia' brought me to tears.

After two weeks of the best sport in the world, marred by a fatal bomb attack in the middle of one night, I returned to inform my News Director that I would be applying for a year's leave without pay to study the Bible at theological college. 'You what——?' he spluttered. He tried to sound supportive yet had clearly been hit for a six. It's not a common request in television newsrooms.

So in 1997, liberated from the constraints of TV, I grew my hair to collar length and spent a marvellous year as a full-time student. It was challenging, unrelenting, high-end theological study that included learning the original language of the New Testament, ancient Greek. Learning a language was also a first for me, but a delightful and enthralling discipline.

The year was punctuated by the death of my father in September 1997 after a heroic two-year battle with cancer. I visited him and my mother most weekends at MacMasters Beach. They were constantly amazed and amused at this new student in their lives. They deserved some payback for all their anxiety over my lack of work during my school years. It provided some much needed relief and a good excuse for a chuckle during those very tough months.

At the end of my studies I gained a Diploma of Bible and Mission and returned to work at Channel Seven as promised. I went straight back into front line reporting and planning for the Sydney 2000

Olympics. As well, with all the new theological knowledge crammed into my brain, I was eager to take on what was already a packed-out year of speaking commitments.

Just two months later the viral hepatitis hit. There would be no reporting, no speaking and not much of anything else for more than two years.

CHAPTER 3

'Just Get Over It'

Monday, 13 April 1998, 4.30 p.m.

After four months of wrestling with the mystery of my health, Meredith and I found ourselves in a surgery at Sydney's Royal Prince Alfred Hospital for an appointment with a specialist immunologist, Dr Robert Loblay. For a number of years he had been a prominent researcher and author of papers on 'fatigue states'. He had established a reputation as a leader in the field in Australia and internationally.

I now realise how privileged we were to have such early and easy access to him. Channel Seven's medical correspondent, John D'Arcy, had pleaded my case with Dr Loblay and organised the appointment. He accompanied us out of friendship and a curiosity to know what on earth was going on with my health.

Dr Loblay began by taking an extensive medical history both before and after I suffered the viral hepatitis in January. I repeated for him the specific and consistent symptoms I had reported to my GP: each day would begin with that feeling of being run over by a truck; my whole body ached like a bad dose of the flu; through the day I would be hit by wave after wave of 'crashes', the worst always coming in the late afternoon and leaving me so ill I had to go to bed, drifting in and out of sleep. I was often desperately hungry, yet despite eating more I was down to my lowest weight in twenty years. I noted especially how an injection of food—even a simple apple or a bag of potato chips—made a world of difference to how I was feeling. (Significantly, I would often say to Meredith, in the wake of the trigger of viral hepatitis, 'Perhaps there's something wrong with my liver.')

Overall, I told him, my body and brain felt like they were running on empty. It was much more than being tired—I well knew how to overcome that. I had spent twenty-five years juggling all sorts of deadlines, time zones and logistics in the news business.

I also explained that part of this feeling of running on empty was suddenly being unable to cope well with stressful or difficult circumstances. It was as if my fuse had been considerably shortened. Often accompanying this inability to cope was a marked tightening of the lungs. I was thoroughly convinced this shortened fuse was a symptom of whatever was going on in my body, not a cause, and Dr Loblay concurred. I also reported some fogginess in my brain, often jumbling words and phrases—I once called our dog, Georgie, 'Jesus'—and a few times putting items of food in the cupboard instead of the fridge.

Another bizarre yet very evident change was a chronic inability to cope with the cold. It was now April and the weather was starting to cool. I was piling on up to five layers of clothing and still freezing. People were frequently taken aback if they felt how cold my skin was.

It was all very puzzling—even more so because, despite a consistency in the symptoms, no two days were the same.

Dr Loblay faithfully recorded every weird aspect of what I was experiencing. In particular, he asked me how I felt in myself—how I was coping with this major upheaval in my life. This was something of a paradox. Despite significant physical suffering and great uncertainty, frustration and distress, I actually felt a strong sense of confidence, purposefulness and security. The basis of this was my conviction that whatever was going on in my body, God was still in control of my life and circumstances and working for my good.

At the end of this extensive and complex summary, Dr Loblay said, 'You give good history.' At least my skills as a reporter had so far remained intact!

He recommended that I embark on a low chemical 'elimination diet', free of additives and flavour enhancers. He also advised me to take up swimming again—until now I had felt too ill and weak to even think about getting back in the pool. He asked me to keep a daily journal of what was happening to me physically. Following my earlier well-intentioned yet disastrous efforts to return to work, he further advised me to take another complete month off and get as much rest as possible. Finally, he urged me to set clear limits in how I managed my life and what I attempted to tackle.

I found this last prospect very hard. At the slightest hint of any turn for the better in my health, my mind would race ahead about the possibility of leaving the illness behind and returning to life and work. I would push myself with any fleeting sign of increased physical capacity, often to my rapid detriment.

The truth was that I urgently, desperately wanted to get back to normal life. I well remember watching a scene in a Harrison Ford movie where he was sweating profusely from physical exertion. How I yearned to be able to sweat like that again!

I enthusiastically embarked on the elimination diet in the hope that therein lay the key to unlocking my health again. Meredith and I faithfully read all we could on the thinking behind the diet and applied ourselves to giving it our best shot, believing it was probably a good thing for everyone in the family to follow.

I also resumed my feeble attempts at swimming—just a few laps at a time. The shock of the cold water was like torture, but I wanted to give myself every chance of getting better.

Sadly, as the days went by, I still woke each morning feeling smashed, and still frequently spent the day shell-shocked. The daily crashes and my growling hunger continued—once the kids heard my stomach grumbling from the other side of the kitchen. Each crash left my body feeling toxic. My sensitivity to the cold grew worse and worse. We all continued to suffer from the shortening of my fuse— at one stage eight-year-old Sophie summed it up with the comment, 'Boy, you sure have to be perfect with Dad these days!'

I could not believe how weak my body had become. In only a few short months I had gone from being able to power through a two-kilometre swim and a session of weights to being exhausted by just a couple of laps. One night, my eleven-year-old daughter, Johanna, beat me in an Indian arm wrestle!

A month after our first appointment we reported all the latest developments to Dr Loblay. He was remarkably thorough in his questions and record keeping, yet at the end the only label he could offer was 'post-viral fatigue state'.

I felt enormously ripped off. How could I possibly be experiencing so many clear symptoms and such suffering, not to mention the mounting losses in my life, and it be nothing more than a 'state'?

Dr Loblay's conclusion added to the suggestions of a couple of concerned friends that I was suffering from 'chronic fatigue syndrome'. Frankly, I didn't want to know about it. A 'syndrome' seemed worse than a 'state'! The idea of chronic fatigue repelled me. I had only ever heard chronic fatigue syndrome described as 'yuppie flu'. It had dodgy written all over it—a mysterious and ill-defined condition that provided a questionable excuse for people to cop out of work or life.

I needed a much more defined label, something real and believable. There was nothing suspicious or dubious about what I was experiencing. I was dismayed at the prospect of being thought of as a bludger or a nutter when I knew I was neither. I certainly had no reason to want to cop out of work and life; indeed, I had everything to live and work for—both now and into the foreseeable future.

One of the reasons I was so desperate for a label was the growing undercurrent among some of my friends and extended family that something more than the physical was going on in my life. After four months people were asking things like 'Do you think it might be mental?' and 'Should you go for some counselling help?'

Some spoke of it as an 'emotional illness'. When one visitor came to see me and I mentioned how much I'd been gaining from a book written by the great nineteenth century theologian C.H. Spurgeon, he replied, 'Oh, do you know he suffered from depression as well?'

In the vacuum created by the lack of a specific diagnosis, people indulged in all sorts of ill-informed speculations. Links were made to the grief I might have felt having to return to work after my year at college. Maybe my long career in a stressful job was the problem. Perhaps I feared returning to the pressures of front line television reporting. There was also my father's death to consider. Could it all have become too much?

I knew very clearly what was going on in my mind and how my faith was keeping it strong despite the mounting suffering and loss. I was also keeping purposeful and organised within the limits of each day. Notwithstanding some mental fogginess, I had by now embarked on a daily program of theological reading for a correspondence course and was continuing my study of ancient Greek. All this kept me occupied and positive, even within my significantly limited physical boundaries.

Yet I found I repeatedly had to explain the very real physical symptoms of what was going on in my body in an attempt to justify myself to people who had already made up their minds about what was happening. Before long I got very tired of it all—and eventually very angry. More and more I struggled with a sense of legitimacy, in addition to the very real struggle of the illness itself.

As the toll mounted on my body, so did this 'collateral damage' of people's attitudes. Each week that went by seemed to confirm the belief of some that whatever I had was more in the mind than the body. People would often remark, 'You *look* good . . .'—always leaving the sentence unfinished as if to say, 'so what's really going on?' Eventually I started to shoot back, only half jokingly, 'I'll hit you if you say that again!'

Always their reply was, 'Well, you *do* look good!' What was I to do?

One unhelpful acquaintance remarked, 'If it was me, I'd just get over it.' I took it that he thought my illness was some kind of lifestyle choice I had made. If I was not 'getting over it', I must have chosen to be in it! That made me rage inside. If only I could transmit just one hour of my physical suffering to such people! Then they would really know what it was like and how impossible it was to 'just get over it'.

John D'Arcy also occasionally wondered aloud about depression—although he acknowledged that if he sent me to a psychiatrist, I would come back with a note asking, 'Why have you sent this man to me?' To help John deal with his musings, I agreed to go onto a course of antidepressants. They had no impact on my physical state. If they had any effect at all, it was to take the edge off my daily desire to keep myself organised and applied to my reading and language study. Ironically, they began to take away my motivation and focus. Now that *was* depressing! I quickly ditched the drugs.

Both John D'Arcy and Dr Loblay were tremendously supportive and understanding in the midst of this great mystery. Dr Loblay especially affirmed the physical reality of what I was going through and kept on wisely stressing the imperative of setting limits, managing and pacing my body and my life. He agreed that the sense of purposefulness and confidence I demonstrated day to day, despite an entirely uncertain future, was a sure sign that I was not depressed.

Unable to see a clear way ahead, Dr Loblay ordered a new series of tests. These set me on a merry-go-round of specialists that continued for the next six months.

I pressed him to sketch out what lay ahead and he urged me to consider re-thinking my future entirely. If this 'state' continued, it could be three to five years before I was out of it. Even then, I would be doing well if my health returned to 80 per cent of what it was before.

For quite a while we investigated the possibility of multiple sclerosis. Just before the 1996 Atlanta Olympics, I had come down with a sudden and inexplicable 'optic neuritis' in which I lost the vision of my right eye. Eventually only 50 per cent of vision returned. Optic neuritis is frequently an early presentation of MS. However, every test returned 'normal' or near to normal.

Over the coming months I was bumped on to four other specialists. With each one the weeks ground on, waiting for appointments and results. This process forced me to come to grips with the large gulf that was opening up between the person I used to be and the circumstances in which I now found myself. My job had enabled me to summon up all kinds of interesting and high-flying people with a simple phone call to be interviewed for that night's news. Now I was forced to endure the whims of doctors' receptionists and the notorious unreliability of overloaded specialists—just like everyone else.

Each new specialist sent me off for a new range of increasingly rarefied tests across a broad spectrum of diseases: cancer, pernicious anaemia, lupus, haemochromatosis, vasculitis, spondylitis, Sjögren's syndrome, Addison's disease and polymyositis.

One appointment stands out in particular. In an already severely debilitated condition, I was tested for a particular muscle enzyme. As part of the investigation, a needle was inserted into the major muscles in my arms and legs and escalating bursts of electricity were fed through it. With each burst my muscle would contract violently.

Poor Meredith was there watching my shock and agony. As she held my hand, I felt her palms perspiring with anxiety. At one stage the technician said, 'Would you mind not contorting your face because it's giving us a false reading.' So I had to sit impassively while he shocked the living daylights out of me.

I shuffled out of the room with a new and powerful insight into what torture must be like. It left me shell-shocked for days. And once again the test result came back: 'normal'. Terrific!

Always, with the mention of a new track of investigation, my hopes would rise that we were finally getting somewhere. Still I lacked a 'label'. I remember well when one specialist rang with a result slightly above normal. I was jubilant—even though this particular condition pointed to a likely early death! My spirits soared that at last we might have some clarity, that this 'thing' was real. Yet over and over again my hopes were dashed and we came up empty-handed.

I often shared my frustrations with John D'Arcy. He remarked about his specialist friends, 'I dare say they probably find you "interesting".'

For nearly half a year now the Seven Network had been very gener-ous and long-suffering with my circumstances. Whenever I had contact with my bosses, they were reassuring and would say and do whatever they could to assist me in returning to health and work.

However, there is a limit to everything. The day before the end of the 1998 financial year, when my contract was due to expire, my boss rang to say they could not pay me any more. It was a bit of a shock, though not unexpected and entirely fair.

My boss insisted that as soon as my health returned they would love to have me back. From this I took it that I was now on leave-without-pay until the day I hopefully turned the corner. So when over the next week a couple of cheques arrived in the mail from work, I was mystified and rang to inquire what they were. 'Oh, weren't you told?' the accountant replied. 'You've been terminated and we've had to pay out all your leave entitlements.' *Terminated?* It was a term that put my life and future into an entirely different zone. It seemed so final.

My first thought was naturally about our loss of income. My boss assured me that under my superannuation insurance policy there was a provision for 'income replacement' in the event of long-term illness or disability. Assuming I met ongoing criteria, this ensured we would be paid a proportion of my old salary for a set period of time. However, he warned it might not kick in for some months, so I had best pursue welfare support from the government.

This became an insufferably long, humiliating experience. Again it was an entirely new world for me. I had long reported on the deficiencies of the welfare system and the difficulties faced by the unemployed, never imagining in a million years that one day I would be counted among them. It was especially humbling to have my name called out at our sickness benefit appointment and for a couple of people to clearly recognise it from television. Character building!

This was an extremely worrying and stressful time. At one stage it seemed that for a period we would receive no income at all from either welfare or insurance. Our trust in God to look after us was tested acutely.

However, in the first week of unemployment, the Lord's Prayer came to me on five different occasions—in a couple of letters people wrote, in a tape I was given and in two books I was reading. One phrase, 'Give us today our daily bread', powerfully penetrated my mind. A book I was reading explained that the original Greek carried more a sense of 'Give us, for this day only, our daily bread'. Jesus' thought was that we should come before God each and every day to seek his provision for our needs. The author made the stunning point that this shows, first, how vulnerable our default state is—something I was feeling acutely! Second, it shows how God can meet our needs every day.

This was perfectly timed to speak potently to our circumstances. In the midst of great anxiety about how we were to survive, we felt God was leading us powerfully to take things one day at a time. We were comforted to know that we could face our vulnerability, certain in the provision of the Great Provider. On many days to come, that sense of security gave us courage to press on.

In the end, our needs were met every single day. Often this happened in unexpected ways, like when we reluctantly cancelled a range of activities in which our children were involved. Amazingly, with each one—tennis, ballet, music and other commitments—'scholarships' were suddenly invented to ensure our kids did not miss out. The private high school attended by our two older children offered us half-price fees. We were profoundly grateful for such amazing and humbling generosity.

After a few months and much mucking around, the matter of the insurance was settled and I was completely extracted from Channel Seven. My payout enabled us to pay off our house, leaving us free of that significant financial burden for the leaner years ahead.

Extracting myself mentally and emotionally from media work was not so neatly accomplished, however. I understood Dr Loblay's advice to pace myself and manage my health, but I really struggled with the demands of the complicated process of extracting myself from work and becoming a welfare recipient.

I felt particular pangs when Meredith returned my work pager and mobile phone and a colleague came around with a small cardboard box of bits and pieces that represented the remnants of my decade-long career. My desk at work had already been cleared out and taken. One night I saw a news promotion on television in which I would usually have featured but was now nowhere to be seen.

Still, there was not one day when, with even the slightest feeling of improvement, I didn't imagine that I could get back to the news business again. The idea of being a chronic fatigue sufferer continued to repel me. I was not an eighteen-hour-a-day-in-bed person, as I imagined chronic fatigue sufferers to be. I could still go for a slow walk each day. I could still go to the pool, though the effort and especially the cold were torment. While my brain had become a bit foggy, I could still manage a fair amount of reading and pursue my love of ancient Greek.

As the days passed, I gradually began to develop strategies to manage my body better. Significantly I started to take food supplies with me if we had to go out for something special—an apple or a packet of chips. These always made a very tangible difference and fuelled me enough to meet the demands of the occasion.

With my constant crashes and severe hunger, I often noted in my journal my conviction that 'something has surely changed in my metabolism . . . perhaps I'm diabetic'. This too I reported to the doctors, who asked if I was ever thirsty, the classic sign for diabetes. I said no. A glucose tolerance test was ordered, but it too returned a reading of 'normal'.

As the spring of 1998 arrived, I tried venturing out into the garden when my body was up to it. I found even a bit of sweeping invigorating. Yet without fail I would take on too much and pay a heavy physical price, often for days.

To my great shock, I also discovered a flip side to my chronic inability to cope with the cold. As the seasonal temperature started to rise, I found the heat was even worse. It produced an intolerable rush of flu-like symptoms—awful aches, pains and crushing fatigue flowing through my body. Again there was nowhere for me to be but bed.

Over and over again I got caught in the heat and was amazed at the physical deterioration it quickly wrought. On one particular walk in the sun, a woman clearly in her eighties with a walking stick passed me!

All through this time, family life had to continue, though often under very different circumstances. With four children aged eight to sixteen, ours was a busy, bustling family requiring a great deal of juggling when it came to logistics, relationships and issues. Much of it was beyond me.

There was never any doubt in my immediate family about the reality of my illness. It was in their face every day!

Meredith suffered much loneliness from having to turn up to events and occasions alone. She also felt the loneliness and frustration of not being able to deal with everyday matters as easily as we had before. My patience would run out too quickly, and the cost to both of us of dealing with difficult issues and decisions was often too great to bear. So lots of stuff was put on the back burner.

She would often say, 'You're here, but you're not here.'

She also became fed up with having to explain our saga to so many people, especially my lack of progress. Too often they would ask how I was going but not think of asking her about how she was. In her 1998 Christmas letter to friends, she reported how much she missed having a vigorous and helpful husband around.

I also grieved at not being an active part of my children's lives. I yearned to take them to a football game and be normal in a thousand other ways. They had to adjust to a much quieter life at home because 'Dad is in bed again'.

One Sunday afternoon I will never forget. Our oldest daughter, Amy, was learning a new piece of piano music and was making the same mistake over and over again. With each of her new attempts, I felt my body spiralling down to a new level of distress. It was truly appalling.

Towards the end of that year, young Sophie suddenly asked me, 'Dad, what will you do in the Sydney Olympics?' I said, 'I won't be at Channel Seven any more, even for the Olympics.' In her innocence she asked, 'Where will you be? What will you be?'

Her questions were like a dagger in my heart. I had no idea where I would be, and *what* I would be was even more of a mystery. Yet it was clear I was no longer the father I once was and still yearned to be.

At Christmas time 1998 I watched from home as the Channel Seven chopper, with Santa on board, landed at the station two kilometres away for the annual children's Christmas party. This had always been a special treat for our kids, making so many of the challenges and difficulties of television worthwhile. It suddenly seemed a world away, and I mourned that our kids were unable to be part of it any more.

After that the family set out on a Christmas camping holiday with me at home in bed. As they left, Sophie crept up and said simply, with tears welling in her eyes, 'Please come.' Who would ever deliberately choose a life like this?

I finished my first year of illness none the wiser about what 'it' was. How fiercely I yearned for some kind of clarity or label!

One specialist told me a story that had particular resonance for me. A woman who had suffered significant ill health for three years without a diagnosis came to see him. In the end he discovered cancer of the pancreas—undoubtedly a death sentence. But her overwhelming response was one of relief and gratitude that at last she had a label and wasn't going crazy. I knew how she felt.

Although all this was pretty bleak, I was still taking comfort in the fact that after twelve months I was managing to remain occupied, organised and purposeful—even though my boundaries had become very confined. Notwithstanding the nagging speculations of too many that this was 'in the mind', my mind continued strong and my outlook confident.

In particular, day after day my personal resources were restocked as I read the Bible, experiencing the same reassurance and comfort that untold thousands have found in it over the centuries. One day this came from Psalm 73:26:

> My flesh and my heart may fail, but God is the strength of my heart and my portion forever.

Another day, there was this from the Old Testament prophet Isaiah, who spoke of a God far larger than I had appreciated before:

> For my thoughts are not your thoughts, neither are your ways my ways,' declares the Lord. 'As the heavens are higher than the earth, so are my ways higher than your ways and my thoughts than your thoughts. (Isaiah 55:8–9)

Although my sense of confident self-sufficiency was being shaken to the core, God always seemed to be there to fill the void. The apostle Paul recorded God's words in 2 Corinthians 12:9:

> My grace is sufficient for you, for my power is made perfect in weakness.

and Isaiah again wrote:

> . . . those who hope in the Lord will renew their strength. They will soar on wings like eagles; they will run and not grow weary, they will walk and not be faint. (Isaiah 40:31)

From my reading I slowly began to gain a new perspective on the wilderness I was in. Again and again, the Bible records how God uses the experience of the wilderness to shape people for the better. Some of the greatest figures in biblical history, like Abraham, Moses, David, even Jesus himself, knew the wilderness intimately. Sometimes I had a strange sense of being privileged to be in this different zone of life—as if I could learn things here that I couldn't learn anywhere else.

My body, however, felt ruined. Much later, John D'Arcy told me that he returned home after one particular visit and said to his wife, 'I think he's dying.'

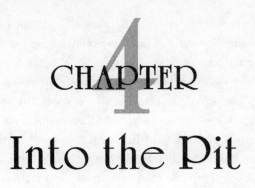

CHAPTER 4

Into the Pit

Wednesday, 27 January 1999, 7.30 p.m.

I entered the second year of my illness in the Sleep Unit of a Sydney hospital. This marked the beginning of a series of significant setbacks in both my physical and psychological health.

I was now on what seemed to me an increasingly futile merry-go-round, wrestling with smoke. One year on, the whole process looked like doctors playing darts blindfolded—and still no one could pinpoint anything that was actually wrong with me.

As part of this I was sent for a sleep test to see if any abnormal sleep patterns lay at the heart of my physical condition. As with so many other tests, the results showed no clear link to my illness. In the end, the only thing the sleep test achieved was to deny me a decent night's sleep. A complex network of wires on my head and chest was hooked up to a bank of monitors. After a horrible night, I emerged the next morning a wreck. It was the last thing my already debilitated body needed.

I went into a physical spiral from which I would not emerge for another six weeks. The flu-like aches were more intense, the crashes more frequent and deeper. The heat of summer left me reeling. I felt as if my blood was somehow poisoned. I spent more and more hours in bed, a few times wondering if this was what it felt like to be dying.

As my physical and by now my psychological difficulties worsened, one particular image kept playing out in my head. It was from the Bible's story of Joseph, made famous in the musical *Joseph and His Amazing Technicolour Dreamcoat*. Joseph, the favoured son of a wealthy ancient eastern patriarch, had eleven jealous brothers who threw him into a pit and left him for dead. I felt as if I was in that pit with him. I imagined a freeze-frame of Joseph in inescapable darkness and contemplated what it must have been like for him. How abandoned he must have felt!

However, the story didn't end there. Though people deserted Joseph, God did not. In the end he was taken out of the pit, and through a long journey with many twists and turns, ended up becoming the prime minister of Egypt and forgiving his tormentors.

I clung onto the full picture of how Joseph's story unfolded, hoping and trusting that the same God who rescued Joseph would one day set me free from my pit.

Although my boundaries were now more restricted than ever, I was still working to occupy myself and remain as purposeful as I could. Facing a new year with a blank and unknown future, I set myself the task of learning ancient Hebrew, the original language of the Old Testament. This may seem bizarre, but I had so loved ancient Greek that I thought tackling another new language would give each struggling day at least some sense of direction.

I also joined a chronic illness support group called 'Hesed', after the Hebrew word for 'loving kindness'. The members became precious fellow-travellers. In the midst of misunderstanding and mistreatment from others, they became an anchor of common sense and equilibrium.

All these new friends bore their trials with grace, graciousness and a surprising degree of humour. They confronted their life-threatening or severely debilitating illnesses with an inspiring confidence in God and a profound sensitivity to others. I found it compelling that one member of the group, who suffered terribly from multiple sclerosis, expressed her dismay at what it must be like living with all the misunderstanding of CFS. The group coordinators often spoke of how much they as healthy people learnt by just sitting back and listening to us chat about our journeys.

Hesed was based at a friend's church, yet each member of the group would often say that, shockingly, church was one of the hardest places for them to be. Sadly, I knew what they meant. More than twelve months into the illness and six months after losing my job, the church office was still calling me to see if I could take on speaking engagements. Somehow the message about the seriousness of my illness was not getting through.

Meredith was also becoming more and more raw from the constant question, 'How's Leigh?' There was hardly ever any new answer to give—no breakthroughs, no developments. Only rarely did anyone recognise the suffering and loneliness that she herself was going through. She had such a burden to bear—so many juggling balls to keep in the air.

It was both surprising and disappointing to me that some of the most upsetting examples of misunderstanding and misjudgment came from a range of people within the Christian community.

In the wake of the sleep test, I was already at my lowest physical ebb to date, and with each new week at church I felt more and more damaged. I hated facing the constant undercurrent of questioning and doubt about the reality of my condition. How I yearned for many of our churches to get their almost singular focus off growth targets, formulas and corporate strategies and to recognise they minister to *people*, especially when it comes to caring for the sick and suffering. As my illness progressed, I was only able to turn up to church about once every three weeks.

I must say with great gratitude that there were many who

faithfully prayed for my family and me. I firmly believe God answered those prayers—not necessarily in making me well immediately, but in keeping me steady and confident in the face of physical suffering and great uncertainty about the future.

However, again and again I would walk away from church having sustained at times significant collateral damage. And many visits at home, though no doubt well intentioned, were too often unannounced, too long and devoid of any real comfort or help. I was often struck by how little people had to say—only things like 'C'est la vie' or 'I guess we can't be much help to you'.

For a long time I had been unable to muster the physical resources to stand up for myself. This had left me vulnerable, alienated and angry. I felt like a boxer in a ring with my hands tied behind my back, forced to accept anything and everything that was dished out to me.

With the physical and psychological harm to my health mounting, at last I felt I had to express my sense of disappointment at how unhelpful and often inappropriate much of my Christian community had been. One year on, they finally began to get the message of how tough the entire experience had been. They responded by organising a working bee of a few young people in our garden and sending a casserole around once a week. We were tremendously grateful. Simple practical help was of immeasurable value.

It is important to add that throughout my illness there were always a few who demonstrated much love and acceptance. One in particular was a man named Maurice Boxwell.

Maurice had devoted much of his life to translating the Bible in Papua New Guinea. From my own study of ancient Greek I had gained a deeper appreciation of the Bible's relevance and power, so I wrote to him acknowledging what an important work he had done. He rang back to express his gratitude, and being aware that I had been ill, asked if he could visit.

As we talked, it became clear that he had travelled much the same road with his health some twenty years before, when there was no notion of 'chronic fatigue'. It cost him four years on the mission field.

Maurice became a precious companion in the following months. He visited every couple of weeks—always phoning to see whether a visit was appropriate, always understanding, always listening and accepting. He never tried to second-guess what was 'really' going on with my health but simply met me where I was. He was a source of immeasurable wisdom, strength, encouragement and practical help.

Some six weeks after the sleep test, I began to emerge from its physical after-effects. I returned to my original specialist, Dr Loblay, still with no formal diagnosis. I was now achingly desperate for some kind of clarity about what had already cost me so dearly. I needed to find my bearings.

After a long consultation revisiting the specific physical realities of my illness, he at long last gave me my much sought-after label: 'chronic fatigue syndrome'. It was the diagnosis I had long expected and resisted, but it was reassuring to at last have something specific to cling on to.

Formal medical definitions of CFS say a patient must have severe chronic or relapsing fatigue for at least six months and must demonstrate a range of flu-like symptoms, including muscle pain, multi-joint pain, headaches, tender lymph nodes, sore throat and unrefreshing sleep. It is often brought on by some sort of viral or other infection. Most of this clearly fitted what my body was going through.

Yet the diagnosis was also perplexing. Uppermost in my mind was a picture of CFS patients as people in bed for up to eighteen hours a day, only ever able to take a few steps at a time. Although I was clearly ill and had experienced much physical suffering, it was never to this extent. I was still managing a short walk around the block each morning and a couple of times a week put myself through the agony of a few laps at our local pool. I was still doing some private study every day. How could I be a chronic fatigue sufferer?

I soon realised that I had been taken in by an inaccurate media perception of chronic fatigue syndrome. Dr Loblay reassuringly talked us through the wide range of possible symptoms and the widely varying degrees of impact. Yes, some people spent eighteen hours a day in bed, but many dealt with CFS at other levels. In one case he related, only two people in the world knew that a particular sufferer had CFS—his wife and Dr Loblay. This man's job took him to various workplaces throughout the day and he was able to sneak off for a rest when he needed to, unknown to his colleagues. I thought: what a burden it must be to bear such physical illness silently, always fearing you will be 'found out'.

I kept pushing for clarity—how long? Dr Loblay said it might be another ten years before I was back at work full time, and I should begin to get my mind around the fact that I would probably never return to the media. He urged me to start thinking laterally about what kind of life and work I could carve out for myself into the future. I said that I had recently seen a bus for the disabled—maybe I could drive a vehicle like that. He suggested I needed to think more in terms of being one of the passengers than of being the driver.

Dr Loblay's sketch of the future seemed grim, but Meredith and I were tremendously grateful for his honesty, clarity and wisdom. He did his best to help us deal with what he well knew was a bamboozling and unpredictable illness.

He encouraged us strongly to take some tough decisions about managing life. Management, he repeatedly said, was the key. It was important to come to grips with the reality of the illness and adjust everything accordingly: expectations, activities, even relationships. Although it seemed as if a sentence had been passed on me, we went away realigned and reassured, with a new sense of direction.

We stopped at a nearby cafe for dinner and bumped into

someone we knew who had heard I was ill. At last I had something to tell him! What an overwhelming sense of relief I felt in being able to say, 'I'm suffering from chronic fatigue syndrome.' I finally had my label.

In the coming days, my twenty-five year media career seemed to fade before my eyes. I set about clearing out my desk at home and a few old boxes of keepsakes. Memories flooded back of times of achievement and purposefulness—memories of London, Canberra, Adelaide and a decade as an on-the-road television reporter. There were lots of old newspaper clippings of a career on the rise and a rich array of security passes and accreditation documents from major conferences, conventions and sporting events around the world.

As I listened on radio and television each day to the excitement of preparations for the Sydney Olympics, I realised I was now totally out of the loop, with seemingly no chance of returning to the inner circle. I felt the loss like a stab in the heart.

I also felt loss about my family. I grieved that I was no longer able to be the person who got dressed for work each day and was seen each night as one of the main players on the nightly news bulletin. I felt the loss of the company car and especially the mobile phone and pager. I missed the departures at the airport and the enthusiastic welcome home at the end of gruelling overseas assignments. I missed that Friday night feeling—being tired at the end of a busy and pressured week, and revelling in the relief of a weekend off. Now, I just felt permanently wiped out without the old buzz of an adrenalin rush to justify it.

I felt entirely diminished both professionally and personally, unable to provide for my family as I always had. I had become a poor husband and father, no longer interesting and involved. I was detached, irritable, stressed out and often in bed. When a friend from Melbourne visited us, how I grieved to see him tossing Sophie, now nine years old, around in our pool.

On one of my morning shuffles around the block, I saw our seventy-year-old neighbour setting out on his spritely daily walk, vigorously stretching his arms to the side and above his head. I felt like I was the seventy-year-old—or ninety!

All my feelings of inadequacy and loss came to a focus in one simple episode at home. The floor of our en suite bathroom shower had been leaking for some time and had finally reached the point where it just had to be fixed. I felt entirely unable to take on the job of arranging the repair, yet I didn't want the responsibility for this too to fall on Meredith's shoulders.

There was a stand-off. She grew more and more frustrated about the worsening leak but was sensitive not to heighten my deepening feelings of inadequacy. I, who had once run logistics that could nearly move mountains, now could not muster the wherewithal to make a couple of phone calls to get quotes for a repair job. I was almost paralysed by inaction.

A couple of times Meredith tried to help out, which only made me feel more inadequate and guilty. On the other hand, whenever I tried to intervene, it would cut across things she had already taken care of. We were barely communicating. The whole thing became an absolute debacle, with a hapless bathroom repairman in the middle.

Some of our closest friends were now beginning to notice our pain and turmoil. One kindly rang the Chronic Fatigue Syndrome Society to inquire about support groups. She gave us the details of their meetings and insisted that we go to at least one.

When Meredith and I first went along it seemed an entirely foreign experience. Neither of us felt we belonged there—or probably more accurately, neither of us *wanted* to feel we belonged there. However, as we settled into the rhythm of conversation among about twenty people, we felt more and more affirmed and comforted in the reality of this baffling illness.

One thing in particular struck me: here were people suffering from chronic fatigue syndrome who were able to be up and about, even if in a very limited manner. It was another important step in breaking out of the mind-set that CFS simply confined the sufferer to bed for most of the day.

We listened carefully to what people said about the practical ways they were managing their lives and health. Dr Loblay was right—management was definitely the key. Our fellow-travellers had clearly found great benefits to their health in making tough decisions about how much they took on. Often these decisions also extended to how they managed the people in their lives. All reported the same shocking abuse from insensitive speculations and expectations.

Discovering I was not alone in this was the greatest gift I could have received. We left the meeting, reaffirmed and re-equipped to face the difficult days ahead.

Whether I was feeling encouraged or dismayed by my contacts with other people, however, there was one constant that never failed to strengthen my resolve to keep going. The God of all comfort was still lovingly at work in my life. It almost seemed that the lower I went and the darker the pit became, the more he was there.

I had a notable experience of this at the very time when my sense of being under siege was deepening.

One day I spent nearly an hour sitting in our backyard with a visitor doing what I continually felt under pressure to do: justifying myself. This time I worked hard to explain the specific physical realities of chronic fatigue syndrome—the flu-like aches, the chaos in my digestive and metabolic systems, the feeling of blood sugar crashes, the extreme hunger, the dramatic loss of weight. There was such fatigue, such weakness and so much sleep. At the same time, I spoke confidently, as if from the core of my being, about how strong I felt in my mind.

As I laid all this out, I remember rejoicing inside that at last I had found a form of words that adequately gave voice to the physical realities of the illness.

My visitor seemed to follow me and connect with what I was saying. When the time came for him to go, he said he wanted to invite me to a particular event. But then he added something strange: he wasn't going to tell me when it was on. He would ring me the day before, in case I 'psyched myself out of going'.

How my heart sank! He had obviously not heard a word I had said. Despite my new-found form of words, he too clearly believed it was 'all in the mind'. As so often before, I felt ripped off, furious and alone.

However, I was not alone. After he went, I logged onto my email for the day and came across what I can only describe as a miracle. On this day of all days, there was an email from a former colleague whom I had not seen or heard from in years. He now worked as a newsreader in a television station in Washington, DC. As far as I was aware, he could not possibly have known about my illness. Importantly, he was not a Christian. Yet attached to his email was, of all things, an animated Bible verse:

For God has not given us a spirit of fear, but of power and of love and of a sound mind. (2 Timothy 1:7)

A sound mind! I was stunned. Here was a powerful reminder of what I knew to be true—that my illness was nothing to do with my mind. I had quite simply fallen ill on a specific day with a specific organic illness.

Although most of the world seemed to think I had lost the plot or was a lunatic, the words of the Bible had yet again given me steel in the backbone—at exactly the right time.

In the wake of the bathroom episode, however, and with the damage I was continuing to sustain from people's misunderstandings, I had to confront the fact that I was becoming depressed. How ironic it was that all the uninformed and careless speculations about my mental state had become somewhat self-fulfilling. Notwithstanding the handful of people who still stood with us in gracious acceptance and love, I was feeling increasingly alienated and angry.

I was also feeling the need to follow Dr Loblay's advice and do something proactive to better manage my life. For too long I had felt powerless and vulnerable, at the whim of others who had their own mistaken ways of dealing with my circumstances. Something had to be done to bring an end to this relational fallout, and at last I was coming to realise that I was the only one who could do it.

A friend at my Hesed group advised me to 'guard my heart'. I had to take on ownership of my health and do what I could to guard it. Acknowledging the spiral I was in, not only physically but also psychologically, I determined to do two things. First, I would write to the two primary pastoral visitors and ask them not to visit any more. This was a very painful thing for me and certainly for them. It was a very great pity it had all come to this. However, too much damage had been done and I felt strongly that I had to take some control of my situation.

Second, I again decided to yield to the occasional yet persistent nagging of my GP and give antidepressants another go. When I tried them the previous year, they had virtually no impact at all, at least on my physical health. Though I remained fully convinced that the cause of my illness was not depression, I recognised it had now emerged as a consequence. I thought it a wise course of action to give the drugs another go—especially for the sake of my long-suffering family.

To my shock, I found I had still not reached the bottom of the pit.

The medication hit me like a sledgehammer. I quickly plummeted off into zombie land. The impact was much greater than the medication I had tried the previous year. These were chronic days indeed—the worst fatigue, the worst pain I had suffered so far.

I spent much of each day in bed, feeling as if I was drifting in and out of consciousness. Sweet Meredith would come in and simply stroke my hand, and all I could offer back was a groan. It was a terrible, terrible time for weeks.

There was certainly no improvement in either my physical condition or my psychological health—quite the opposite. What physical strength I had took a sharp dive, and the familiar symptoms of debilitating fatigue and that overall toxic feeling were exacerbated. I often felt as if I was in some kind of twilight zone of suffering and unreality. The few things that had kept me focused and occupied, like my Hebrew and reading, rapidly evaporated.

When I first reported the distressing consequences of the medication to my GP, he was almost excited that there had been such an impact. Perhaps, he wondered, we were onto something at last. I could hardly believe what I was hearing. He even entertained increasing the dose!

It all came to a head about six weeks later. The antidepressants had intensified the already considerable difficulties I was having with my digestive and metabolic systems. One Saturday morning, while the rest of the house was sleeping in, I rose and went to the toilet. Without warning I was hit by an overwhelming wall of pain in my gut. I had never experienced anything like it in depth, intensity or suddenness. I struggled to return to the bedroom and passed out on the family room floor. Meredith heard the thud and came rushing out. She picked me up and helped me towards the bedroom. There I passed out again. The agony was unbearable. I blessedly made it to the bed where the pain vanished as quickly as it had come.

Poor Meredith was in such a panic she rang 999 instead of 000. Next she tried my doctor, who rushed around. He was clearly rattled by what he saw. We had a long talk and I unloaded all the ways in which the antidepressants had made my health and my life much, much worse. I decided again to take on greater ownership of my health and insisted that I be taken off the medication. He had no choice but to agree.

There began another month of out-and-out physical collapse as my body and brain were realigned off these powerful drugs. I had reached the bottom of the pit at last.

CHAPTER 5

Flickering Light

Monday, 16 July 1999, 3.00 p.m.

The first flickering light at the end of the tunnel nearly slipped by without my noticing. In the broad sweep of the illness it was almost imperceptible. Indeed, it was only when I looked back over my journals to write this book that I could clearly see the tentative and faltering beginning of the end.

It happened on the day I got a haircut.

By the middle of my second year of illness, such a simple outing was quite an undertaking. I dreaded the cost to my health of any move out into the world. I also dreaded the inevitable chit-chat of a hair appointment which may sooner or later turn to my health. I was at such a low ebb psychologically that my confidence was shot to pieces, and the prospect of running into more misjudgments about CFS and having to justify myself yet again was almost too much to face.

After fuelling my body with an apple I arrived but nearly turned back as I walked in the door of the shop. It all seemed so daunting.

As I feared, the conversation with Tara, the hairdresser, eventually led to the question, 'And what do you do?'

'Well, nothing much,' I answered. 'I'm ill with chronic fatigue syndrome.'

I braced myself for the usual reply. But to my utter astonishment and enormous relief, Tara said she knew all about it—her brother had suffered CFS for years. When I explained how it had all started with viral hepatitis, she said that her boyfriend had suffered a weird hepatitis/malaria-like condition two years before and his health had never been the same since.

I had already learnt that there were only two kinds of people able to truly understand and accept the reality of chronic fatigue syndrome: those who had suffered the illness themselves and those who had seen a close family member suffer it in their home. I regarded Tara and her ready acceptance and understanding as a real gift. At last an outing beyond the confines of home and bed had not left me in worse shape. Free of a mop of hair, and for once free from misunderstanding, I remember how good I felt as I walked out.

The very next evening we went to the house of some friends for dinner, along with another couple. We discovered that the husband in this couple had lived with CFS for more than a decade. For the second time in as many days, it was liberating to be with people who could give me acceptance and understanding. They also offered a breadth of wisdom on day-to-day management and setting limits. They too recounted heart-wrenching stories of what they had suffered through years of people's doubts, judgments and ignorance. Meredith and I deeply appreciated their quiet acceptance of their predicament, and their determination to make what they could of a limited life.

They had worked hard to figure out why there was so much misunderstanding about CFS. The explanation they proposed was called 'the myth of idleness'. Most people, they believed, see a life of idyllic idleness as the ultimate yet unattainable indulgence. Healthy people often imagine that the long-term ill have attained this goal and resent them deeply for it. When an illness like CFS emerges with no specific medical marker, there are constant doubts about whether sufferers are really ill or merely indulging themselves. If only people who think this way knew how boring idleness quickly becomes—and how CFS sufferers yearn to get on with a life of health, vigour, productivity, decent relationships and usefulness!

Once again, we went away from that night reaffirmed and re-equipped to 'keep on keeping on'. The slight improvement in my health had lasted another day.

Two things happened as a result. First, as usual, my mind raced away with all the dreams and plans of what it would be like to be well again and have this awful saga behind me. Second, I immediately put my body to the test.

I could sense the first taste of spring and my love of gardening beckoned. As I set about transplanting a couple of roses, I was shocked at how weak my body was. Still, it was exhilarating to get out and engage in even a small amount of physical exertion.

Unfortunately, it all turned out to be fleeting. Before long my body crashed—severely—and I was flat on my back in bed again.

The roller coaster ride intensified with this brief yet tantalising taste of something approaching normality. I grasped hold of it as confirmation that I had not been conning myself into illness or conning others by taking on the 'myth of idleness'. My spirits had soared at one fleeting ray of light—even though, in what seemed like the blink of an eye, the light had been snuffed out.

From that time on, however, a faltering pattern began to emerge. Every two weeks or so, I had one day, or perhaps even two, when I felt a discernible improvement in my health. I sometimes woke refreshed instead of feeling as if I'd been run over by that truck in the middle of the night. My body had slightly more staying power through the day. Sometimes I even escaped one of the constants of the previous eighteen months, the late afternoon crash.

Every time this light dawned, without fail, my mind would race ahead planning a future without illness and I would push my body too far to another inevitable crash. I then tried to pace myself more wisely and better manage any improvement, in the hope that it would last longer. However, time and time again I couldn't help myself and pushed myself over the limit and over the cliff.

This pattern of one step forward, one step back continued for months. There was no accounting for the improvement. It was as bewildering as the illness itself.

One thing I was increasingly certain about, however, was the impact that food had on how I managed the day. Since my first year of illness, I had been fuelling myself with a piece of fruit, a bag of potato chips or a sandwich before any outing. It always gave my body more to play with, even if only for a short time.

This food–health connection now became more and more obvious. I remember starkly a visit from a friend late one afternoon. This was almost always my 'red zone' when the only place for me was bed. She brought some sashimi to share and I could not believe the difference it made to me. It held off the all-too-familiar crash and enabled me to engage in conversation in ways that reminded me of my old life pre-illness.

Time after time, quite inexplicably, food was the thing that enabled me to keep going for just a little bit longer. On the other hand, some foods, often heavily laden with fat, sent me on a rapid downward spiral.

As this challenging new chapter was opening up, a friend told us of a university lecture by a visiting overseas professor who specialised in managing those with long-term illness. Fuelled by my fruit, I went along with Meredith to hear him speak.

His talk was compelling. He unwrapped the notion of being both a 'pilgrim' and a 'nomad' in facing sickness over the long haul. The constant challenge, he explained, was to keep a balance between being on the pilgrim's journey with a sense of direction, and being forced to live the life of a nomad, lost in the wilderness. Of particular help to me, he affirmed how difficult and painful was the constant struggle for legitimacy. He also had lots of good advice on accepting the new person that illness had forced me to become and the limited life I now led.

We were especially heartened to see Dr Loblay in the audience. He was clearly someone who was always seeking to be better informed about the issues of long-term illness.

We had already booked to see him one month later. He asked me a surprising question: 'What would you do with your life if you had cancer?' My immediate and instinctive response—no doubt shocking and offensive to cancer sufferers—was born out of my struggle for legitimacy: 'I'd be relieved!' But his question was aimed at forcing me to confront a life that would continue to involve significant restrictions and narrow horizons.

As so often before, I wondered aloud whether I could ever entertain thoughts of resuming a career in the media. I had begun to think of perhaps setting up my own media business to gain more control over how I worked and for whom. Time and time again, two potential avenues of work came to my mind. The first was the fledgling twenty-four hour Pay-TV news channel Sky News Australia, which had recently hit the airwaves. The second was the Bible Society, an organisation I had already had some limited contact with.

Again Dr Loblay said I should probably ditch such ideas and find some limited form of activity I could engage in without significant cost. He had given this advice many times before, but this time his prediction of recovery taking years hit me with new force. It really did appear that my career in the media was at an end. I guessed that my hope of resuming my work on the speakers' circuit was also finished.

We retreated to a small Indian restaurant nearby for a meal. I was speechless—not depressed or despairing, just overwhelmed at how different and unsure the future suddenly seemed. I had lived a life of activity, purpose and usefulness, and in my mind I had always been determined to get through this illness and resume that life. How could I begin to think of living an absolutely minimalist existence? The notion seemed utterly foreign—such an intrusion into so many plans and dreams. For nearly two years my body had been saying 'no' to a life of activity. Now I had to get my mind around dealing with it for perhaps the next decade.

One thing Dr Loblay dealt with helpfully was a persistent feeling of guilt that both Meredith and I had experienced. This came from the pressure we felt from people's urging us to 'do something' to get over or around the illness. Dr Loblay insisted that, although there were no drugs to take and no more tests to undergo, we were actually doing a great deal by devising physical and emotional management strategies. We needed to keep on refining what worked for us.

Notwithstanding this excellent advice, we continued to feel the weight of people's expectations. With my specialist saying my health might remain in this pit for years, I struggled more than ever to know how to answer all those who kept saying, 'You *look* good . . .' I developed one form of words: 'Today I'm OK—I'm managing. I spent the first six months finding out where my limits are, the next year respecting them, and now I'm managing them—most of the time.' Ninety-nine per cent of the time I could have saved my breath.

The problem was this: if people wanted us to 'do something', which one of the endless and diverse options should we choose? Acupuncture? A never-ending range of expensive vitamin and dietary supplements? Alternative medicine or natural therapies? Cold bath therapy, anti-allergy medications, antimicrobials, anxiolytic agents, more antidepressants? The list of possibilities went on and on.

No one realised the amount of psychological capital Meredith and I had invested in the various tests I had undertaken or how emotionally depleted we were when it came to considering this diverse range of alternatives—none of which had been recommended by Dr Loblay. One day Meredith cried out in despair, 'You can't even do anything to help yourself!'

Around this time an interesting and ultimately highly significant couple reappeared in our lives. We had briefly known Peter and Penny when we lived in South Australia fifteen years before. Peter was a doctor working in Adelaide.

Now we discovered that Penny had been suffering from chronic fatigue syndrome for the past six years. Her illness was so acute that she had spent much of that time in bed. There were occasions when the weight of a watch on her wrist would prevent her lifting her arm. Because of Penny's illness, Peter had developed a kind of mini-specialty in his medical practice dealing with numbers of CFS patients. He was also aware of some significant research into the illness that had been underway in South Australia.

The four of us began to engage by phone and email. As with Dr Loblay, Meredith and I went away from each conversation empowered and affirmed to press on.

From the research it appeared that, for some unexplained reason, some chronic fatigue patients were not able to metabolise enough energy for their cells. This had a particular impact on the brain, which uses so much energy. Peter explained that the body, and especially the brain, shuts down under these conditions as a kind of protective mechanism. Hence the wide range and diversity of symptoms involved in CFS.

Peter came to visit us when he flew to Sydney for a conference. I explained my occasional good days, but he urged me to treat them with great caution. 'By all means make the most of them,' he said, 'but don't push so hard that your body once again throws up its arms in surrender.' He said he looked for three to six months of consistently good health with no relapses or setbacks before he would pronounce someone well again.

I felt his advice gave me permission to enjoy the good days but not abuse them, and not to get overly excited about kick-starting my life again the next day. He agreed with Dr Loblay on the time scale—seeing it had been nearly two years already, we were probably looking at a long haul.

Still feeling the weight of expectations to 'do something', I asked Peter what he would advise. He said research and his own clinical experience had shown some benefit in vitamin B-12 injections—one injection a week over three months. He cautioned against seeing this as a 'magic bullet'. But it was something that was reasonably benign and would bolster my body's defences. Perhaps it would give me a little more health to play with.

I was happy to take his advice, though I did so more than anything to appease those urging us to be more proactive.

I went for my injections to the nursing home where Meredith worked as a physiotherapist. A kind friend there had offered to give me the weekly jabs.

As she threw the first one in, she said, 'Now I can say I've jabbed a celebrity.'

I replied that I thought those days had gone.

I felt that at last I was beginning to get my mind around that reality and accept it. Just a couple of weeks before we had a new television aerial fitted on the roof of our house, and I remarked to the workman, 'I used to be on television.' It was the first time I'd said anything like that to anyone. It seemed such a landmark.

But making this transition was very painful. In fact, I was now grieving the loss of my old career as never before.

At this time, one of the biggest stories in Australia's region exploded off our northern coast in Timor. An overwhelming vote for independence from Indonesia was being thwarted by pro-Indonesian militias. The situation rapidly descended into a bloodbath, and grave tensions emerged between Australia and Indonesia. Teams of Australian journalists and news crews, including many of my former colleagues, rushed to report on a story that was quickly taking on all the appearances of a war.

I learnt that even John D'Arcy, my work colleague and unofficial medical advisor, had gone to Timor. How I yearned to be there with them all, adrenalin rushing and in the middle of the action!

Instead, the biggest thing in my life was a decision I had made to weed our back lawn. As the crisis unfolded over the coming weeks, I followed it on my pocket radio while sitting around our yard and laboriously digging out buckets of weeds. Instead of the thrill of the story chase and the sense of achievement and purpose, each day for me was measured in squares of weeded grass.

When a former work colleague visited and cheerily declared, 'Maybe Timor will swing your mind back into getting better', I nearly despaired.

Around the same time I drove one of my daughters to the Aquatic Centre that was to be used in the Sydney Olympics. It was nearly two years since I had seen it. As the Seven Network's Olympic correspondent, I had reported on the very first construction work at the site, then followed it all the way through to the centre's opening. But for nearly two years I had lost all contact with Olympic construction.

Returning for the first time, I was awestruck to see the broad sweeping boulevards, the marvellous sporting facilities and the monolithic Olympic Stadium. I was now resigned to the fact that I would miss all the excitement of the Olympics, certainly from the perspective of my old job. I guessed I would also miss being a spectator, unable to afford either the tickets or the physical toll of such an outing.

I remember standing there drinking it in with tears welling up in my eyes.

I am bound to report that for the first month of the vitamin B-12 injections, my health took a turn for the worse. I can only imagine that the vulnerable state of my body simply could not handle anything new, no matter how benign. The serious crashes returned and the occasional good days were snuffed out.

My frustration deepened towards those who so flippantly made us feel as if we weren't 'doing something'. Every time I embarked on a new proactive course I hit a wall. Through that first month I returned to the days of feeling completely smashed from the moment I woke up. I spent long days in bed in significant physical pain. The limited range of activity I had tried so hard to maintain, such as the few laps at the pool, was curtailed.

Then, again almost imperceptibly, the odd good day began to return. Most days still brought the same old flu-like aches, the fatigue, the toxic feeling through my body, the inability to cope with either stressful situations or temperature variations. However, every now and then, I would clearly have more capacity—not a great deal, but more than usual.

Two highly significant things happened by the end of those three months of vitamin B-12 injections. First, I put on weight—about seven kilograms. Something had clearly changed in my metabolism.

Second, out of the blue, I won an Indian arm wrestle rematch with my daughter Johanna—the one who had thrashed me just one year earlier. This time I beat her with no great effort.

I was on cloud nine! A victory at last!

CHAPTER 6

Hasten Slowly

Thursday, 21 October 1999, 10.10 a.m.

I opened the front door of our home and offered an encouraging greeting to my visitor: 'You've lost a fair bit of weight since I last saw you.'

'And you've lost a fair bit of hair since I last saw you!' he shot back.

Greg Buckley was a master of the quick, quirky one-liner. It was a joy to see him again. I had first met him eleven years earlier when our circumstances were entirely reversed. He had no way of remembering that first meeting, or a number of subsequent encounters.

Back in 1988 Greg was a tall, strapping nineteen-year-old on a fast track to the big time of Rugby League and the bright lights of fame.

In the late afternoon of Friday, 5 August 1988, he was playing in a President's Cup Rugby League match. It was being televised. In the final stages of the first half, the video shows the ball being fed out along a line of players until the play is switched and the ball is passed to Greg. He is tackled by two players. The first grabs him around the knees and he begins to fall to the ground. The second player, just as he's falling, hits him with a tackle to the side of the head. It has the effect of whip lashing his head to the ground. His head bounces once and his whole body collapses to the turf—seemingly lifeless.

All the doctors say Greg should have died that night, or during any one of the days that stretched out afterwards into weeks and then months.

The Monday after his fateful match, I began working in the Seven Network's Sydney newsroom as a senior reporter. Greg's story was one of my first assignments. As he hovered in a coma between life and death, I was asked to see if his parents would talk to the media. I pursued a number of avenues and understandably no one from his immediate family was in any state to talk. I chose not to push it. Weeks later I made another gentle approach and there was still no reply.

In fact, unknown to me, they were checking me out to see if I had the sense and sensitivity to be able to deal with a shattered family and a young man still at death's door. Out of the blue they rang and said I had the story on my own. The rest of the media was still being held at bay.

When I first saw Greg in the hospital he was brought in strapped in a wheel chair, with a feeding tube protruding from his nose. He was conscious, but only just. He had no reaction to the television crew. The lights were on, but no one seemed home. It was shocking to see his condition.

In the coming weeks, through several stories, I established a real connection with his family. Slowly he regained his life over the next few years, but still with some permanent brain deficit. As his recovery progressed, I went back and reported on a number of major milestones. I covered his first day back at college, resuming his training to become a nurse. Then there was the triumph of him learning to drive and ultimately his graduation from nursing college—a most moving event.

Eleven years on, the tables were turned. Greg, now married with two children and working as a nurse educator, came to visit his ailing reporter—with an offer. He had heard that I was ill and thought I needed a project to 'get me going again'. He wanted me to write a book about his story.

Right from the outset he refused to take no for an answer. He had lived through much of the previous decade smashing through the many seemingly impenetrable walls of brain injury. Words like 'no' and 'never' had long been blown out of his vocabulary.

After a marvellous chat catching up on all the events of the intervening years, Greg left fully convinced that his book was underway. I very much doubted it.

By now—October 1999—I had experienced several months of having one good day every couple of weeks. After the initial shock of the vitamin B-12 injections, my body was marginally changed in a number of ways. The severity of the daily crashes had eased somewhat and I had regained some of my lost strength. I continued to have many more bad days than good ones, but there was still an occasional flash of light.

Hope began to stir yet again. I came across one striking statement in the book of Job, that classic story of great suffering and God's sustaining power. It expressed my longings exactly: 'For there is hope for a tree, if it is cut down, that it will sprout again, and that its shoots will not cease' (Job 14:7). How I longed for this to be me—for the occasional glimpses of light at the end of the tunnel to be the dawn of a new life, free from sickness and suffering.

As the end of 1999 approached, my marginal improvement enabled me to embark on a few more outings. These included the end-of-year Christmas carols night at our children's high school. That night I was enthralled by one thing: the organ playing that accompanied the singing. The organist was a highly regarded musician and teacher who also happened to be a school mum. My mind was filled with the richness, power and beauty of her playing.

I left the service captivated by the possibility that I might use my little bit of extra health to learn to play the organ. I had learnt piano as a child up to fifth grade, and had resumed playing over a decade earlier when we bought a piano in Adelaide. Now that I was gaining the odd day of good health, it might be a way of taking on something positive and enjoyable to push those small gains a little further.

For several days I became totally preoccupied with the possibility of learning the organ. I contacted the woman who had performed at the carols service to see what she thought. She agreed to help me out, even within my limited boundaries, and said there were a number of churches in our area with fine pipe organs that would be happy to allow a student to use them. This was all wonderful news.

I was not at all certain how my body, and especially my brain, would stand up to the challenges of learning music again. It is important here to draw a distinction between my brain and my mind. I knew my mind was strong, yet my brain so often felt as if it too, like my body, was running on empty. I had already completed a number of units and even exams in my theological correspondence course, pacing myself through units of Greek, Hebrew and church history, scoring in the 70 and 80 per cent range. But would I have the capacity to engage in the complex, demanding task of learning the organ?

I didn't know. However, I was convinced that my desire to take on this challenge was another potent practical demonstration of the strong state of my mind and my heartfelt desire to be out of the pit. If only my body were as strong and resilient as my mind. All too often my body would draw a clear line in the sand.

Sadly this also happened with my dreams of becoming an organ virtuoso. Reality struck only six days after the carols service. Sophie came bouncing home from school with a new clapping rhyme she had learnt. She was eager to teach it to me. It was four o'clock and I was entering the day's 'red zone'. To a quite shocking degree, the more she tried to teach me the song and the clapping routine, the more my body went into a rapid spiral. Rarely had I felt my brain emptying so quickly, as if someone had pulled a plug. My whole body went into a kind of toxic shock that sent me reeling.

As I lay in bed, stunned by the suddenness and severity of the decline, I was forced to confront the grim reality that my brain as well as my body was not up to the challenge that my mind was getting so excited about.

I also felt fury as I realised once again that I had been conned into thinking a positive new mindset or activity would simply kick start me back to health. Over and over, the mistaken notion that I had chosen this new life had driven me to try to prove the doubters wrong. I kept on trying to push myself through the wall of CFS, but always ended in more and more physical trouble—an intolerable price of suffering piled upon suffering.

As the vitamin B-12 injections came to an end, we yet again faced the pressure to 'do something'. After what seemed to be hundreds of urgings to try some kind of 'natural therapy', we decided to follow one particular lead from an old friend of ours. She had suffered CFS and had been in the care of a GP who also prescribed naturopathic therapies. These treatments and naturally occurring substances are said to stimulate the body's own healing abilities.

Frankly, I was not at all convinced of their worth, but I decided to give them a go for no other reason than to be seen to be 'doing something'. I was comforted in this case that the alternative medicine was being advanced by a conventional medical practitioner.

The doctor took an extensive case history of my illness and at the end posed an interesting question: 'What was going on in the lead up to all that?' I described the period leading up to the episode of viral hepatitis that triggered the whole saga two years earlier. I gave her a comprehensive run-down of my job, family, the death of my father and my year of full-time study at theological college. She too was convinced that the state of my mind and my level of even limited activity precluded all notions of depression. Her conclusion: 'There's no doubt you've got all the manifestations of chronic fatigue syndrome.'

Her main advice was based on the old saying attributed to Caesar Augustus: 'Hasten slowly.' She ordered a full blood screen and gave me some green stuff to drink, along with some white powder that we jokingly referred to as finely crushed monkey testicles. She recommended a course of vitamins, especially vitamin C. Her aim was to deconstruct the individual components of CFS and address each symptom in specific naturopathic ways.

The blood screen test came back with one hardly surprising result—I had been overdosing on vitamin B-12. The doctor said it would take months to dissipate.

The coming weeks continued to provide about one day in every fortnight of better than average health, frequently blown apart by my infuriating propensity to overdo even the slightest improvement. The bad days were as bad as ever. Christmas Day 1999, with all the chaos, calamity and noise of our family gathering, was a disaster. It was all intensified by the inevitable delays in Christmas lunch. I ended up rushing too much food into my mouth too quickly, being driven out of the kitchen by a flurry of women in the midst of frantic preparation. It only served to send me into a sharper spiral. It was an absolute shocker for which I paid a high price over much of the coming week.

Greg Buckley continued to badger me about writing his book. I did my best to hold him at bay, trying to explain how fragile and unreliable my health was. In fact, I twice told him 'no'. He refused to accept my feeble pleadings. Eventually I caved in, unable to hold back this dogged steamroller. I set clear and specific ground rules that I would only embark on the project subject to my health standing up to it. It would be an unconventional and, I suspected, sporadic endeavour.

Meredith too was not entirely convinced of the wisdom of taking on the project, but she did make one passing comment: 'I'm sure we'll look back on Greg's re-emergence and say, "Wow, wasn't that interesting timing?" '

I can't say the naturopathic therapies made any noticeable difference to the overall state of my health. I gave them my best shot— anything to gain some sort of improvement.

As much as anything, I benefited from the wisdom of my naturopath GP, who focused on treating 'the whole person'. She urged me to use the benefits of the sporadic good days for my healing, not to waste them on the world. She explained the concept of 'banking' the good times and not frittering them away. It all sounded so sensible, even if I found it impossible not to grab hold of any improvement and physically, as well as psychologically, go for broke.

As the year 2000 got underway and I approached the two-year mark of my illness, we had a few days away at the beach where it all started. Watching my kids frolicking in the surf, I was suddenly struck by how much I had lost since that summer of 1998.

In that snapshot of time it was not the loss of my job, future plans or even health that hit me hard. It was the fact that it was me, of all people, who was stuck on the sand while everyone else was enjoying the freshness, fun and foaming waves of the beach. In my former life, wild horses could not have kept me out of the water. Now, my general health, and particularly my body's acute aversion to the cold, kept me stuck on the sand, looking on wistfully.

The other thing that cut me to the heart was how much older my kids suddenly looked. I had lost so much of the past two years of their lives, never to be regained. How I grieved that loss.

Early in the new year I received three interesting and entirely unrelated phone calls, seemingly out of the blue. One caller asked whether I would consider hosting a weekly half-hour interview program for Anglican Television. Another, from an independent video producer, asked whether I might be available to present a corporate video he was directing.

I instinctively and immediately declined both offers. Such commitments were at this stage entirely out of the question. However, I told both callers that I was beginning to see the first flickering of light of what I desperately hoped would be a turning of the corner. Maybe a little further down the track I could dip my toe back in the media pond.

The third call came from a former radio colleague I had not spoken to for nearly twenty years. He had likewise suffered significant periods of ill health and been forced to organise his personal and professional life around illness. He had managed to carve out a viable and fulfilling work life from home, writing, consulting and conducting occasional workshops in media training. He was convinced that, with the experience gained in our line of work and our extensive 'contact books', every journalist 'was walking around with a million dollars in his head'. That, he implied, included me.

What on earth was I to do with all this? I was still surprised to think I had agreed to write my first book—and now these tantalising and exhilarating phone calls suddenly popped up. Help!

Of course, any notion of jumping back into the media was against all the best medical advice I had received for just on two years. Call me foolish, stubborn, pig-headed, thick—but in reality I still could not accept the idea that my media career was over. Some of my old colleagues clearly thought I had reached the end of the road: one friend said she was out at a bar with a group of Channel Seven journalists when my name came up and the conversation suddenly fell embarrassingly silent. 'It was as if you had died,' she said. And there was little else to encourage me—I could not even say that I was steadily getting better and better. Yet as long as there was the odd day of clearly better health, I had enough to cling to and hope for the best.

Then came the most significant phone call of all. It was our friend in Adelaide, Penny, who had suffered chronic fatigue syndrome for six years. Her doctor husband, Peter, had come across some ground-breaking research that pointed to the metabolic system as the area that needed to be addressed for some CFS patients. On the strength of that, he had sent her off for some heavy-duty tests to look at her blood sugar and insulin. For once, the tests came back with significantly abnormal levels.

He immediately put her on a diabetic diet, although she was not diabetic. She began eating more often, and eating food that would sustain her body for longer. She was also steadily and carefully increasing her level of exercise.

Penny was riding high on the difference it was making in her life. She was now out and about in the car, cooking the evening meal and basically getting a life again. She was not back to 'normal' or to what she used to be, but she reported a remarkable turn-around.

I immediately booked an appointment with my naturopath GP to see what I could do with Penny's experience. She too was tremendously excited, and kept saying over and over again, 'It makes heaps of sense.'

It definitely made sense to me. Perhaps the 'blood sugar crashes' I had tried in vain to explain to everyone were exactly that—blood sugar crashes. Perhaps, after all, my body and my brain *were* running on empty. Perhaps this was why I had always felt the enormous benefits of food, and why my few feeble laps in the pool each week always left me feeling better for the next twenty-four hours. Exercise is a trigger for the liver and muscles to release more sugar into the blood stream and hence make energy available to the body. Perhaps the original viral hepatitis had in some way damaged or changed the function of my liver, the engine-room of the metabolic system.

My doctor agreed to send me off for a similar three-hour test, looking at my blood sugar and insulin. While she was quite definite that we were still operating under the broad umbrella of chronic fatigue syndrome and not diabetes, I rushed to some of Meredith's old university textbooks to read up on the elements of diabetes. There I found a number of highly significant correlations—the blood sugar crashes, the inability to cope well with stress, fluctuations in the body's temperature regulator, even the benefits of exercise.

For the three days leading up to the test, I had to markedly increase my intake of food. This was both good and bad news. There were ways in which it clearly gave my body more to play with, feeding my metabolism. However, not knowing exactly the sorts of foods I should and should not eat, I found the crashes, when they came, were markedly worse.

How I prayed as I turned up for the blood test that something would be found!

Sure enough, two days later I learnt that my insulin was high. There are no words to describe the sense of relief and unbounded joy I felt at finally finding out that something *was* wrong with my body.

During this time my mother decided to remarry. When her husband-to-be rang with their news, I was tremendously happy for them both.

They asked me if I would read a passage from the Bible at their garden ceremony. By any measure this would be a major outing, so I decided to put all the new information on my illness to the test.

As we left for the hour-long drive to MacMasters Beach, I fuelled my body with an apple, then on arrival went straight for some biscuits and cheese. These sustained me through the ceremony and especially my reading. Rarely before had I felt under such public scrutiny, especially in front of members of my extended family who had seen my illness as more mental than physical. As soon as the ceremony was over, I dived back into the biscuits and cheese, was then sustained marvellously by lunch, and then a sandwich later in the afternoon, normally my 'red zone'. The whole day went brilliantly.

Still somewhat tentatively, I dearly hoped that this was what turning the corner felt like.

I had organised with my mother to mind their house during the week of their honeymoon, for which I set myself three goals. First, I would use the peace and quiet to give myself the best chance of managing my diet, although I still did not really know exactly what I should and should not be eating. Second, I planned to increase my level of physical activity—walks on the beach beckoned powerfully. Third, I would begin in earnest to write Greg Buckley's book.

Undistracted, I managed to get about five hours of writing done each day, broken by a long walk on the beach and a short rest in the middle of each afternoon. Though there were still a few crashes and my body would still go toxic at different parts of the day, I was clearly gaining substantially more capacity and could make much more of each day. Slow and faltering it may be, but liberation was dawning.

A couple of weeks later, I went for a second, longer blood test. I had fasted the night before and drunk a small bottle of a sugary soft drink at 8.00 a.m. Over the next five hours my blood sugar and insulin were tested every half hour. I returned home smashed and gobbled down a couple of sandwiches. My body went into melt-down. The combination of fasting, the short, sharp shock of sugar and the five further hours of nothing to eat, followed by a sudden intake of food, was more than it could handle. I spent the rest of the day and that night in bed in a great deal of trouble. It was another one of those times when I wondered if this was what it felt like to die.

However, in the end it was all worth it. The results came through two days later, confirming markedly abnormal levels in both my insulin and blood sugar. Peter and Penny shared my elation. They knew the feeling well. Peter recommended that I take the test results off to a dietician to see what could be done to stabilise my sugar and insulin levels.

After the experience of my mother's wedding day, I decided to put my body to the test of a regular outing. I had continued to press on with my learning of ancient Hebrew and in the process had heard about a fortnightly Hebrew reading class at a Sydney theological college that was open to anyone interested. Armed with a couple of apples and a sandwich to keep me going through the morning, I embarked on a walk to the train station, a twenty-minute train trip and another ten-minute walk to the hour-long class.

It all went wonderfully. Admittedly, by the time I made it back home I was fairly exhausted—but at least I made it! Furthermore, I paid no great price for this first step out into the real world. I had kept my body fuelled, and with a bit of exercise it did not go into the familiar late afternoon collapse. I committed myself to attend the class once a fortnight, seeing it as an important yet still friendly test of how much my body could be sustained.

As usual, on the back of such success, my mind raced ahead with possibilities. I began to think about how I could translate these tentative but significant gains into work. I knew with certainty there was no way I could commit myself to a full-time job, especially one on the front line of TV journalism. However, perhaps I really might be able to set up my own business at home. I could operate as a free-lance writer and take on other associated jobs. That way, I would have a better chance to pace the demands on my body.

I made a few calls about the corporate formalities of setting up a home-based business, as well as launching out on the odd outing to look at computers, desks and other office equipment. I was admittedly rushing ahead of myself, but these first steps into the big outside world were truly thrilling.

When I went to see the dietician towards the end of March 2000, she looked at the results from my five-hour blood test and said she had seen diabetics with these sort of readings, though she too emphasised I wasn't diabetic. She gave me a wealth of information on what and how to eat, as well as advice on increasing the level and intensity of my physical activity.

As I left she said, 'I have no doubt by the time I see you in two weeks you'll have much more to play with.'

I dared to dream she could be right.

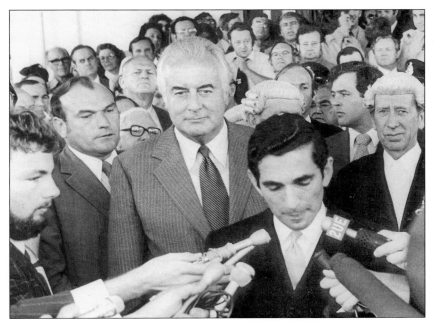

The sacking of Prime Minister Gough Whitlam, 11 November 1975—with me as a bearded young radio reporter on the left.

With a Channel Seven news crew, May 1994.

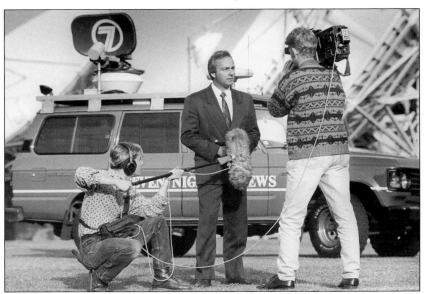

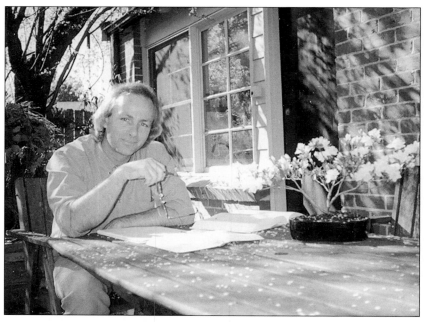

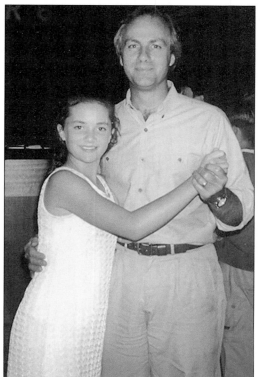

Enjoying life as a long-haired student, July 1997, the year before falling ill.

A rare outing during my illness with my daughter Johanna, who at eleven beat me in an Indian arm wrestle. November 1999.

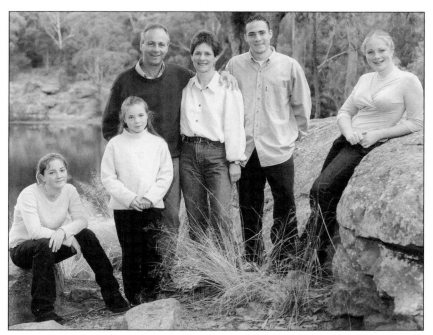

With my family (left to right): Johanna, Sophie, Leigh, Meredith, Tristan and Amy—three months after my health 'turned the corner'. July 2000.

Behind the scenes of Olympic Sunrise, *October 2000.*

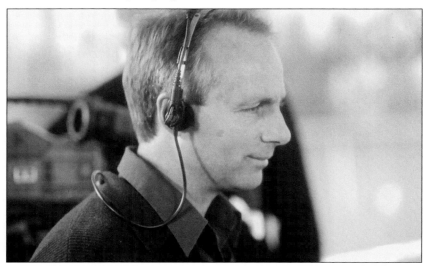

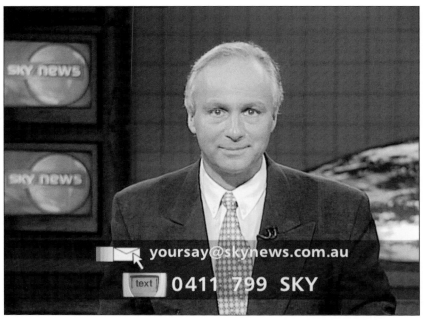

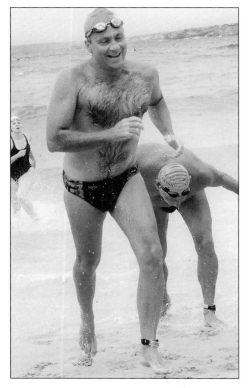

On the set as a news presenter at Sky News Australia, March 2001.

Emerging from the Cole Classic rough-water ocean swim, a major triumph three years after my recovery. February 2003.

CHAPTER 7

Turning the Corner

Tuesday, 23 March 2000, 5.30 p.m.

I left the dietician's office with her words of hope ringing in my ears and a folder of information under my arm. It detailed how I would now live, eat and exercise. The plan was quite simple. With blood sugar and insulin levels approaching the realm of diabetes, I needed to eat and exercise as if I were a diabetic. From now on I would have to eat more often and choose foods that sustained my body for longer periods of time.

Part of the information pack was the so-called 'Glycaemic Index'. This index ranks a wide range of carbohydrates according to the way they impact on the body's glucose and hence its energy levels. Highly processed or sugary foods and certain carbohydrates are at the top end of the index. I was to avoid these because they give the body a sharp shock of energy, then a sudden crash. Instead, I was to eat foods ranked at the lower end of the index. These release energy more slowly.

Such a diet would still allow me to eat a wide and enjoyable range of foods, but I would need to make some fundamental changes. I would need to replace white bread with sourdough or mixed grain breads. I would need to eat more for breakfast, including a bowl of porridge or a cereal high in grains. I would also need to eat something every few hours as a between meals snack, even if it was only an apple with its slow release sugar. I would have to even out my meals more, not packing in a large dinner at night—an overnight crash from a large intake of food in the evening explained why I had always woken feeling so wasted.

Having noticed throughout my illness the difference that eating made, this new information gave me the concrete knowledge to match my suspicions. What had been a random hit-and-miss attempt to help my body get through the day now became a systematic program. I had to adopt a significantly different way of eating, to accommodate the new state of my body.

The dietician's other piece of advice was to increase the amount and intensity of my exercise. This would demand more from my metabolic system and force it to operate more efficiently. It would help even out the peaks and troughs of my body's sugar and insulin response.

I put her advice to exercise into immediate effect. The next morning, instead of my usual shuffle around the block, I pushed myself into a brisk walk. I immediately knocked ten minutes off my usual walking time. Georgie, our dog, who had patiently plodded alongside me on our walks for two years, struggled to keep up with my new-found pace. Within a couple of days one of our neighbours said to his wife as he saw me bounding along, 'Is that Leigh?' By the time she turned around to look, I was gone.

The days that followed seemed like a rush back into life—though tempered by the reality that my body was still different and I was not immediately over it all.

Less than a week after visiting the dietician I tried another outing, this time to Sydney airport to pick up my mother and her new husband from their overseas honeymoon. Driving through the city

I felt a strange and delightful sense of reconnecting with the world. After two years spent moving largely between my bed and our backyard, that simple car trip opened up striking new horizons. My mother was both stunned and thrilled to see me at the airport.

Another day I woke early and seemed to be bounding with energy. On my walk I felt entirely diverted by the sheer joy of living a life again. I went shopping and bought a new pair of shoes and a briefcase, then had a good swim and did some gardening. I still felt pretty tired, but it was *just* tiredness—nothing like the old crashes. I felt such joy, such relief, such a sense of vigour returning.

With my new capacity, I embarked on concrete steps to set up my own home-based business. A friend helped us overhaul and paint the room that would become my office. I set about ordering a computer, a mobile phone and a range of office equipment.

That same week I registered the name 'Omega Media'. I felt like saying to the lady who dealt with the paperwork over the counter, 'Let me tell you how significant this day is!' The name had long been in the back of my mind. It picked up the way 'omega', the final letter of the Greek alphabet, is used in the last book of the Bible, Revelation. Coupled with the first letter of the Greek alphabet, alpha, it is used as a title for God—'Alpha and Omega'—signifying that God is the beginning and end of all things. It also looks forward to the day when God will wrap up all of history and those who are his will be restored and regenerated in security with him forever.

I felt my two years in the wilderness had deepened and broadened my experience of life and God. If I was able to take up any kind of work again, I wanted it to be built on the foundation that the main game lay beyond the pressures and distractions of each day.

Recalling my former colleague's advice that 'every journalist is walking around with a million dollars in his head', I began to reconnect with old contacts. At almost every turn, often in quite stunning ways, this produced prospects for my new business. A neighbour enthusiastically embraced me into his advertising agency for a wide range of writing tasks. I landed a couple of scripts for corporate videos to write, produce or present. None of it was in the broadcast world from which I had come, but the skill-base I had honed in my former work enabled me to branch out into areas I had never dared to tackle before.

I quickly realised that one benefit of working for my own company was the degree of flexibility it would open up in my work life. It struck me how similar this was to what I had planned on that beach, way back in 1994. Then I had dreamt of walking away from full-time work after the 2000 Olympics and balancing freelance media work with some kind of itinerant Christian ministry. Though it had been via an entirely different route, and for entirely different reasons, I marvelled that I seemed to be ending up in the same place.

Two weeks after that landmark visit to the dietician, I had booked a follow-up appointment with her to gauge my progress. That morning I was so pumped at the prospect of reporting my break-through that I cut myself shaving—twice.

I walked in and said simply, 'You've given me a life again.'

She was thrilled, but cautioned me against the rush I was already finding it extremely hard to resist. A 'measured' return to life, work and activity would give me the best chance of building on this major turnaround in my health. I found it almost impossible to exercise any restraint. The shackles of CFS had bound me for so long—how could I not go for broke, even though I was still hitting the odd wall?

Just two days later I embarked on my first work outside the relative security of my home office. The idea came from a former colleague who was working as a freelance media trainer, equipping executives and others with the skills required to appear on the media. I had made an appointment to speak with the managing director of the training company he worked with. I could hardly believe how daunting the prospect seemed. As I got dressed in a suit and tie for the first time in many months, it was exactly like getting ready for my first job interview.

This was my first inkling that a massive crisis of confidence was dawning. It stemmed, not from being cut off from everyday life for such a long period, but from people's constant suggestions, overt and oblique, that I couldn't cope, had stressed out or had some kind of work aversion. You can only be treated like that for so long before you begin to have massive doubts about yourself. I felt like a cowering dog that had been kicked around and hit too many times for its own good.

In the event, however, the meeting was extraordinary. Most amazing was the fact that the MD had an extensive and intimate personal knowledge of chronic fatigue syndrome as his daughter had suffered with the illness. I noticed when I began to talk about CFS that my top lip began to tremble in a nervous quiver—no doubt part of that 'kicked dog syndrome'. He was tremendously reassuring, saying he would give me all the time I needed and every opportunity to pace myself. I was profoundly grateful.

I left the interview with my head spinning. The MD was very keen to put my years of media experience to work. There was even the prospect of interstate and overseas travel with some of his significant contracts. I was to return in four days' time to take my first media-training workshop. It was all very exciting.

Physically, I was now moving ahead in leaps and bounds. I felt like a ball of muscle, revelling in the sheer joy of getting a life again. Meredith would return from an outing and instinctively go into our bedroom to catch up on how the day had gone, but the bed would be empty. I was 'up and at 'em'!

I felt much more like engaging with people again. At a neighbourhood gathering I was able to last and last—and noticeably, to laugh and laugh. With real progress to report, at last I could take the initiative in conversations. No longer did I have to be defensive and on the receiving end, always waiting for the inevitable misunderstandings.

Accompanying all this were some small but for me towering breakthroughs. I mowed the grass for the first time in two years. I shared a picnic with the family on the beautiful shores of Sydney Harbour. Meredith said I was brave, and she struggled to find words to explain the amazing things that were so suddenly happening.

I fronted up for my first media training workshop armed with an array of apples, tubs of yoghurt, fruit bars and sandwiches. It was now about a month after beginning to turn this significant corner in my health.

The workshop was a one-on-one session with a senior public service executive whose organisation had been through a major media crisis. I began with a great deal of hesitancy, but the whole exercise ended up feeling just like the good old days. I had done hundreds, perhaps thousands, of media interviews and putting him through a number of interview scenarios was a breeze. The skills I had built up over such a long time had not deserted me. Despite my anxieties, I had been able to jump back on the horse again.

The rush of work continued. Within that same week I received two offers for which I had a special affection. First, John D'Arcy sounded me out about writing scripts for a medical TV program he presented every couple of months. Over coffee, I met with him and the program's producer and enthusiastically embraced the idea of working with them. It seemed to be challenging and fascinating work, which I could accommodate according to the health or work needs of the day.

Another offer of work came in a call from Tom Treseder, the Bible Society's chief executive in New South Wales. Tom had visited me at home during my illness and had often rung inquiring about my health. He asked whether I would consider producing and presenting a video for the work they were doing distributing Scriptures at the upcoming Sydney Olympics. Over and over again during my illness, the Bible Society had been in the forefront of my thoughts about where I could work if and when I recovered. The Bible had been so critical in shaping, comforting and equipping me over the past two years. Again, I enthusiastically embraced the opportunity.

Within a couple of weeks, the production of this video had me back out at the Olympic Games site. Only four months from the opening of the Games, I was again in awe at how much had happened there. Where once a deserted wasteland and ramshackle buildings had been, immense sporting structures and state-of-the-art facilities were now set to welcome the world's elite sportsmen and women. It was fabulous to have the opportunity to be there once again.

One month after that landmark visit to the dietician, I returned to the Olympic site with my family for the 2000 Royal Easter Show (it had moved to the site just after I had fallen ill). The annual agricultural Show had been a favourite of mine as both a child and a grown-up, but it had been entirely out of the question during the years of my illness. I grieved to see each year's Show pass by with my kids going and me staying home, often in bed. Now I was fiercely determined to make up for lost time, and I had an exhausting, exhilarating day back amongst its captivating noises, sights and smells.

In the middle of thousands of people, we even bumped into my dietician and her husband as we were walking through the agricultural produce pavilion. I had just bought an apple to keep my body fuelled and she was delighted to see me munching on it.

Within a few more weeks I fulfilled another long-held dream, sustained right through my illness—to take my two eldest children to a State-of-Origin Rugby League game. Even more significantly, the match was held in the main Olympic stadium as a trial run for the upcoming Games competition. I took unbridled delight in being able to be once again part of such an occasion. How I had longed to be that kind of father again—to be able to take my kids to the footy!

All this contact with the Olympic site began to sow a tantalising seed in my mind. Could I, despite the grim predictions of my doctors, consider returning to the Olympic broadcast arena and finding a media role somewhere for the two weeks of competition?

I was still not entirely sure about my health or capacity. Though I had made previously unthinkable strides in work and activity, about one day in every two weeks I would still hit the wall as my body went toxic and I was overwhelmed by the same old fatigue. This brought me down to earth with the grim realisation that the saga was not totally over. Yet I had been able to push myself enough to at least consider exploring opportunities for work at the Olympics.

My first inclination was to attempt a return to familiar territory, back at Channel Seven, the holder of the broadcast rights for the Games. It still felt like home to me. The executive producer of Olympic programming, Andy Kay, had been a junior producer working for me more than twenty years earlier when I was program director at Radio 5DN in Adelaide. We had also been in Atlanta together in 1996, enduring all the highs and lows of that marathon effort. I decided to ring him and see if there was any chance of work for the 'Olympic Network'.

I wasn't at all optimistic. It was hard to imagine new staff being put on only a few months out from the Games. I also well knew the enormous physical demands of covering the Olympics and could not say with absolute honesty that I would be physically up to the effort of a Games campaign.

Andy, however, was overwhelming in his response to my call. To my great surprise he said he was certain there would be a position for me somewhere. He said he would call in twenty-four hours. When he did, he had an offer of one month's work covering the two weeks leading up to the Olympics and the two weeks of competition. We negotiated a generous daily fee that would put down a very solid foundation for my new business.

He rang back a few days later saying he wanted to extend the offer to two months' work, such were the overwhelming demands of broadcasting the Olympics on home soil. On the strength of that, I went out and bought a little car for my fledgling business. The demands of work and family were such that already we were running into logistical problems with our one vehicle. These were good problems to have!

I was appointed senior producer on *Olympic Sunrise*, the daily three-hour breakfast-time TV program planned for the week before the Olympics and the fortnight of competition. It would require a very early start, considering the program was scheduled to begin broadcasting each day from 6.00 a.m. On the strength of our previous professional relationship, I felt able to confess to Andy some very real uncertainties about whether I was going to be able to take on the 'Olympic marathon'. He was most encouraging, and over and over expressed his joy at seeing me back in the fold at Seven and in the Olympic Unit.

One thing I felt unable to confess to Andy, however, was the continuing struggle with my crisis of confidence. I was still very much suffering 'kicked dog syndrome'. In fact, my progress out of illness had unexpectedly emboldened some people to come and say things they hadn't felt able to say before.

One person, within a few weeks of my turning the corner, hit me with this: 'I guess it's just like in the Bible when Jesus heals a lame man. The first question he asks is, "Do you want to be well?" I suppose it's that time for you now.' I was flabbergasted. In my still raw state, it seemed to me that yet another person had all along thought my illness was some kind of choice I had made.

How could anyone imagine me to be such a fool as to endure even one hour of what I had gone through—with all the loss of job, esteem and family life—because I didn't 'want' to be well? I knew in my heart of hearts how wrong this was. I knew how enthusiastically I was embracing better health again now that I was finally turning the corner.

Much to my alarm, the collateral damage I sustained from such people continued, despite my returning health. One asked how I was doing, but when I excitedly explained the massive strides I had taken in work and life generally, he pointed to his head and said, 'No, how are you feeling up here?' I felt like hitting him! A few also latched on to the fact that my sudden turn-around had come at the same time as my mother's remarriage, as if getting her off my mind had enabled me to 'get over it'.

It was becoming a monumental challenge to bridge the gulf between the exploding demands of my new work life and the doubts I was continuing to suffer about myself. Somehow I had to come to grips with this crisis of confidence—especially as I was now returning to the 'confidence business'. The one essential requirement for work in the rough and tumble of commercial television is confidence. It is not an industry for the faint-hearted, and certainly not one for those who have 'lost the plot'.

At least most of my job as a producer on *Olympic Sunrise* would be behind the scenes, with only the odd on-air report. To my enormous relief I would not have to do anything live-to-air. I felt completely unable to tackle the demands of that mountain.

There is one particular development to report from this time that seemed to us an out and out miracle. The insurance money that had sustained us through my illness came to an end just as I was beginning to earn a steady though still humble income. The timing was perfect— 'heaven sent'—and I was deeply grateful that we had been spared the huge financial difficulties that I know many CFS sufferers endure.

The week after the money ran out, I savoured one particularly sweet day. I sat on an aircraft ready for take-off to Melbourne for an overnight video shooting job. What delight I took in sitting there with the familiar sounds, smells and sensations of an aircraft cabin. After the long months of loneliness and isolation, I revelled in being among fellow air travellers. I had been here hundreds of times before, but on no other flight had I felt such elation.

As the aircraft rumbled down the runway, I couldn't wipe the beaming smile off my face. Lift off!

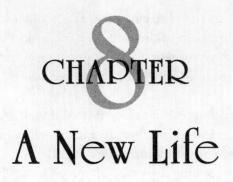

CHAPTER 8

A New Life

Monday, 7 August 2000, 8.55 a.m.

For the first time in more than two-and-a-half years, I walked through the front gate at Channel Seven. Although I had been so much a part of the place for most of the previous twenty years, I now felt like the new boy on the block. I was tentative and uncertain—feeling the very real symptoms of 'kicked dog syndrome'. But it was great to be back.

I walked into the chaos of the Olympic Unit about six weeks before the Opening Ceremony of the Year 2000 Games. It was very scary. There was a palpable sense of an avalanche looming, ready to dump on this frantic and often confused bunch of people.

It hardly seemed possible that they could undertake such a mammoth broadcasting feat in a matter of weeks. No wonder they were still taking on extra people like me.

My job as senior producer for *Olympic Sunrise* was entirely ill defined, as was much of the show itself. It was only four weeks away from going to air. Now that was *truly* scary!

Within a few days I was on another of those flights that had always seemed so ordinary yet were now so thrilling. I travelled to Alice Springs in the red heart of Australia, then to a magnificent gorge of towering red ochre cliffs. It was a highly secretive trip with a handful of Australian athletes to do a story on the new Olympic uniforms they were to wear at the Opening Ceremony. The dominant colour of the uniform was the same red ochre as this spectacular gorge.

During the rush of the shoot, I allowed myself a quiet minute to sit among such grandeur and beauty and contemplate how far I had come in just a few short months.

When I was appointed to the Olympic Unit, all the accredited media places for the International Broadcast Centre at the Olympic site had been taken. I was only able to work at the Seven studios. Considering where I had come from so recently, that seemed more than enough, although it was still a bit disappointing not to be part of 'the main game' where the competition would be held.

Before long, however, it became obvious that my role demanded a daily presence at the International Broadcast Centre. To my surprise and delight I was granted a special accreditation. Having my photo taken for my accreditation pass was another defining moment. It was a small matter but held such significance. I was back in the inner circle of the Olympic movement, about to embark on another Games marathon.

It was terrifying, but oh so sweet.

Pretty soon my job became a twelve to eighteen hour, seven-day-a-week roller coaster. With less than a week to go before *Olympic Sunrise* went to air, we embarked on a few frantic days of rehearsals.

The program's location was as good as it gets—a multi-million dollar, two-storey townhouse on Sydney Harbour overlooking the world famous Harbour Bridge and Opera House. The whole apartment was transformed into a working TV production and studio facility. The large upstairs bathroom was make-up and a bedroom next door was the news studio. Downstairs, another bedroom was transformed into the control room and our editorial office was in the bedroom next door. The lounge room and balcony constituted the main set where the show would go to air.

The first day of rehearsals was a disaster. There were a number of major technical crises, programming content was virtually non-existent, and the logistics of organising such an undertaking in such a foreign environment were a disaster. As we gathered rather stunned for a debrief, we all felt sick. Everyone wanted to walk away, but we had only four days to get it right before we went to air.

The solution was a complete overhaul of how and where everyone in our tiny unit worked. I was assigned a shocker of a shift. I was to start at the International Broadcast Centre at 10.00 p.m., working on pre-production for the content of each day's program. At 3.30 a.m. I would catch a taxi to our harbour-side townhouse and help the presenters, Johanna Griggs and Andrew Daddo, with their preparation. I would then supervise the three hours of the program on location as it went to air.

There was one very special gift in these few frantic weeks. I learnt that Johanna had had her own battle with chronic fatigue syndrome. She had been an Olympic swimmer and lost two years of her life when she came down with the illness in the early '90s. Our journeys out of CFS had been very similar. She too had discovered the huge benefits of eating frequently and eating well, as well as the need for exercise. Jo said she would eat up to ten small meals a day to keep her body fuelled and keep up with the demands of a high profile life. Often as I arrived at the townhouse to prep for the program, I found her already in make-up devouring a big bowl of spaghetti bolognaise—at 3.30 a.m. Our shared experiences and our conversations about what we had gone through were very precious.

The demands of my role on *Olympic Sunrise* were far beyond what I had anticipated, although as an Olympic veteran I should have known to expect the worst. I had to quickly develop a rigorous plan to maintain the diet that had worked spectacularly so far. Each night I brought a pre-cooked dinner and a number of trusty apples and fruit bars. I also took some porridge to cook at the townhouse at 6.00 a.m. each morning as the show was going to air. Each program would end with a bacon and egg roll for the crew at our daily debrief. It all sustained me remarkably considering the severe constraints of only six months before.

With each new day of rehearsals, the program was bedded down. Our new roster seemed to work much better. We all felt that sense of quiet, ominous dread as the minutes counted down to our first show. It could not have had a worse start. By what almost appeared to be evil design, the autocue died the very second the opening theme rolled. Jo and Andrew had to wing it in a moment of sheer terror.

I believe they 'nailed the gig' from that moment on. *Olympic Sunrise* became one of the shining lights in the Seven Network's coverage of the 2000 Games. It perfectly captured the joy and wonder of two memorable weeks of competition and the buzz and joy of Sydney's transformation into the Olympic city.

For everyone on the crew it was a grinding, punishing schedule, and at the halfway stage—as with every Olympics—it seemed like it would never end. The wrap-up of our final show was a sweet moment of triumph. Then there was that declaration from Juan Antonio Samaranch at the end of the Closing Ceremony that Sydney's were 'the best games ever'.

I celebrated at the Olympic Unit's wrap party with my first beer in four years.

I left the wrap party at 2.00 a.m. and swung into my very next free-lance job at 9.00 a.m. the same morning.

In the last week of the Olympics I had been rung by a television producer I had known for years. He was putting together one of the early reality TV programs called *Treasure Island*. It was in the same genre as *Survivor*—two teams trapped on a deserted island—but in this program they were vying to win a treasure chest of money. Overwhelmed by other projects, he needed someone urgently to work for six weeks writing the concluding six episodes of the program. I accepted the offer though I had never taken on anything like it before. It was another steep and demanding learning curve.

In the middle of the Olympics I had received another far more significant call. It was from the managing editor of the relatively new twenty-four hour Pay-TV news channel, Sky News Australia. This was the very place that I had often wondered about working if I ever 'turned the corner'. He said he had heard I was back in the land of the living and wanted to offer me some work reading the news.

'I've always thought if there was one person tailor-made for our operation, it's you,' he said.

I was flattered—and horrified. My work on the Olympics had been largely behind the scenes, with only a little on-air reporting. None of it was live-to-air. Month-by-month my health was taking steady steps up from what had been a most debilitated state, and I had been able to take on enormous challenges and stay upright. But I still felt I had a long way to go before I would have the confidence to take on live air work again.

When I look back on this period now, I see how hard this struggle to regain my confidence was. In some ways it became the most arduous part of my recovery.

I continued to take hits from those who still considered my illness a 'can't cope' disease. As I was taking on more and more work, one of the few former colleagues who had stuck by me throughout the illness remarked as a kind of joke, 'I never thought work was supposed to agree with you.' I wasn't very amused. It wasn't easy to find myself on the receiving end of such ongoing misunderstanding while at the same time taking on—and conquering—demanding jobs back on the media front line.

In a way, I was faced with more than just 'kicked dog syndrome'. I was actually battling to know who I now was. My life had been through an upheaval involving a lot of personal, as well as physical, damage. I now had to prove to myself that I *could* cope and *was* able to handle stress—that I did not have a work aversion. In short, I was struggling to find where I fitted in again.

Without doubt, out of simple human pride, I was hoping for even a tiny bit of recognition of how rough the last couple of years had been and how good it was that I had been able to make it back out again. However, I soon realised that most people expected me just to slot back in where I had left off. This was impossible considering all that I had been through. I found it very difficult to fit back into all the expectations, and especially the relationships, of what I now saw as my former life.

I had gone through a profoundly life-changing experience. It been long and it had been deep. In a number of significant ways it had changed me—I am convinced for the better. I had certainly become a much more compassionate person, yearning to be a comfort and help to people going through life's tough stuff.

In particular, my time in the wilderness had redefined the breadth and depth of my faith. It had vastly enlarged my view of God and broadened my view of the scope of life. I still signed on to all the elements of orthodox evangelical faith, but I had become more and more convinced that God looks more at who we *are* than at what we *do*. It was liberating to be free of all the obligations and expectations that I fear imprison so many in the Christian community. I felt more able now to live a life motivated by love and unbounded gratitude to God for everything he had given me.

I had also come to the dawning realisation that it is very often in the midst of weakness, vulnerability and suffering that God does his greatest work. Something my prolonged illness had exposed was the extent to which my life was based on a mistaken sense of self-sufficiency. It was only when I discovered how vulnerable I was that I really came to appreciate the size and scope of God—to know, in the depth of my being, his mercy and grace.

Reading the living history of the Bible, I saw how unmistakable it is that God sometimes leads his great people of faith through the wilderness, often for a long time. Yet it is there that God reveals himself profoundly. What God had revealed to me especially was his utter trustworthiness. Even when events seemed to be spinning out of control, even when my best laid plans went up in smoke, even when others disappointed me and led me to despair—there was still One in whom I could trust. I now believed that the biggest lesson we can draw from the entire biblical narrative is how God can be trusted, always. And the biggest thing that God surely wants of us is simply to trust him.

None of this ever dawned on me until, like Joseph, I went down into the pit. It completely revolutionised my whole understanding of life and faith.

Unfortunately, it also set me apart from my old Christian community. I felt acutely how sad it was that many people had been unable to come alongside me in acceptance and understanding as I went through this experience. I met several times with the leaders of my church and there were heartfelt apologies for their shortcomings. I readily and wholeheartedly accepted these and felt a genuine sense of forgiveness.

However, in practice, I felt the 'new me' had nowhere to go to have my new insights and understandings affirmed and understood, let alone embraced. I found it impossible simply to walk away from the experiences and insights won in the midst of suffering. They were too real and tough for me just to pack them away in a box and move on as if nothing had happened.

At the end of the day, all this created a significant disconnection from my old stream of church life. For one reason and another, attempts to achieve a reconciliation and accommodation kept on hitting a wall. Sadly, I still found myself feeling alienated, alone and damaged, even in the midst of galloping good health.

Thankfully, my work life continued to flourish, even though here too it was really challenging slotting back into the type of work I had for so long taken for granted. I agreed to go into Sky News Australia to talk with the managing editor about doing some casual news-reading shifts.

I looked around the operation there. Compared with the news-reading jobs I had at Channel Seven, the job at Sky was very much DIY.

At Seven the newsreader was treated like the star, having all his scripts collated, the autocue run by a specifically dedicated operator, a freshly chilled glass of mineral water poured and the microphone clipped to his jacket by the floor manager. At Sky News there was none of that. For a start the newsreader was the only person in the studio—there was no floor manager to shepherd him through the ups and downs of the bulletin. There were no camera operators either—the cameras were run by remote control, like robots. The newsreader was responsible for all the scripts, the (tap) water, the microphone and even the autocue.

As soon as I saw the little accelerator-like pedal under the desk that the reader uses to drive the autocue, I thought, 'I can't do that!'

The other vast difference between Pay-TV news and network news was the sheer volume of work. At Seven I had only ever read one news bulletin a day, with the assistance of a separate sports reader and weather person. At Sky I would have to read every-thing—news, sport and weather—and there was a bulletin 'on the hour every hour', each one lasting thirty minutes. A reading shift consisted of up to six of these half-hour bulletins, going out live across Australia and New Zealand and into Asia. It was a world away from what I was used to.

There was no easy way to regain the confidence I had once known. The prospect of doing live television again scared the living daylights out of me, and the anticipation of taking it on consumed me. Finally I arrived at the defining moment of my first bulletin at Sky—1400 hours on Saturday, 21 October 2000. As with my very first TV bulletin twelve years earlier, I sat there with sweat running down my back as the red light on camera 2 went on and it was me, alone and live. It felt just like starting out all over again.

As is often the case, the anticipation of the fearful event was much worse than its execution. I quickly felt at home again with all the familiar elements of news reading. But there were challenges. Having to read with the constant stream of necessary cues and control room chatter in my earpiece was a colossal mental exercise. There was also the vast amount of reading. For weeks I walked away from each shift in a state of mental exhaustion.

It was a traumatic experience fighting to regain my confidence in the context of such physical and mental demands, combined with the ultimate scrutiny of the TV camera for hours each shift. I remember filling my car with petrol on the way home from one shift and feeling envious of the mechanic pottering away beneath a car. How lucky he was to earn his living in such relative simplicity!

It took a good three months before the strain began to ease and I felt I owned my new job more than it owning me. Yet again, I marvelled that those fleeting yet optimistic thoughts of working at Sky that I had in the depths of CFS had come true.

In the middle of my rush back to work, I had to grab time to conclude the interviews for Greg Buckley's book. It already seemed another lifetime ago that I started this landmark project. Meredith had been right—it had come at just the right time. There was a special place in my heart for Greg and his story, and it was a thrill to present the manuscript to him a year after we began our project together.

It is important to acknowledge that for all the gains I made, my health was not back to what it was before. For the first six months after turning the corner, I moved into each new month noticing tangible improvement from the month before. My body was stronger and my capacity growing beyond my wildest dreams.

By the end of 2000, however, the improvements had plateaued out. There were still elements of each day when I knew my body was different. If it was not fuelled as it should be, or if I pushed myself too hard, I would get that old toxic feeling back again. Notwithstanding the demands of frequent shift work at Sky, I still needed earlier nights, and under the stress of normal home life my fuse was still shorter than it used to be pre-illness.

I was back to about 90 per cent of the health I had known before I fell ill. However, my new life was a world away from what I had known in the depths of CFS.

In time I came to revel in my work at Sky, delighting in the exhilarating highwire act of live television. It became my favourite job of all the varied roles I had undertaken in my three decades of broadcasting.

Eventually one of the studio directors jokingly nicknamed me 'The Grim Reader'. Although each of the newsreaders worked on a set roster system, when a really big event hit in those first couple of years it always seemed to be me in the studio. This began with the events of 11 September 2001, less than a year after I began working at Sky, and went on to include the major bushfire crises that hit Sydney in 2001 and 2002, the Bali bombing, the catastrophic Canberra bushfires of 2003 and the very moment the war in Iraq broke out in 2003, as well as the symbolic end of the war with the toppling of Saddam Hussein's statue in central Baghdad.

With each new big event it seemed the demands at Sky grew and grew. We began to do more 'live and continuous' coverage, running stories on air for hours at a time when news was breaking. At the height of the 2002 bushfires, I ran our coverage for the entire six hours of my shift without a break. Only one hour of it was scripted. I first sat down in the hot seat at noon and didn't get out of the chair until 6.00 p.m. I was surprised how wobbly my legs felt when I finally stood up at the end of it all!

This was incredibly demanding, mentally exhausting and professionally fulfilling work. It was not for the faint-hearted and definitely not for anyone with a stress problem. Although some of the doubters would never be convinced, at least in my own mind I had proved them wrong.

CHAPTER 9

A Fall with Grace

Sunday, 2 February 2003, 10.50 a.m.

One week in early 2003 marked two more highly significant turning points in my journey back. It began on Sydney's famous Bondi Beach on a perfect Sydney summer morning where I lined up ready to dive into the Cole Classic rough-water ocean swim.

Over the previous year I had steadily increased my swimming to five kilometres a week, but only in an Olympic-sized pool. I had never taken on anything like an ocean swim before, primarily due to a lifelong fear of sharks. However, at the urging of a work colleague, I agreed to take my life in my hands and give it a go. Around 2500 swimmers were to take part in the two-kilometre race. I figured I would be pretty unlucky if a shark picked me off out of that number.

I stood alongside 135 male swimmers of every shape, size and ability in the forty-five to forty-nine year old age group. The air was thick with bristling testosterone. My heart was racing as we waited for the starter's signal. Suddenly, in a frenzy of spray and foam, we were off.

Yet again, the anticipation of the event was much worse than the execution. Throughout the race I felt cocooned by other swimmers around me, some passing me, others I was overtaking. Quite a number swam right over me—rough-water indeed. After swallowing what seemed like litres of water, I made it to the finish line in a time of 36 minutes 22.3 seconds. All up, I came 1427th in the race—for me a total triumph.

I emerged from the surf with my limbs intact, not a shark in sight, and in a state of euphoria. While I knew before that I could swim the distance, I was not entirely confident of making it under such demanding conditions. After catching my breath, I stood on the beach with Meredith, soaking up the warmth of the sun and the smell of the salt water, drinking in the moment. For once I was not a reporter of a major event but a participant, and my own personal victory in making it to the finish line was sweet indeed.

We had lunch with some friends, Bruce and Judy Baird. Bruce had been the state government minister responsible for the successful 2000 Olympics bid, and had also taken on many ocean swims. They had become good friends, especially through the long march of my illness. We sat in the warm afterglow of a great Sydney summer event, rejoicing in how I had come this far. I felt it was truly miraculous.

Later that week came the second most significant turning point beyond the turnaround in my health. It concerned my still troubled church life.

A couple of months before, I had finally reached the point where I felt I had no alternative but to move churches. This was a deeply difficult process for Meredith and me. She had been shown much kindness by her close church friends and never experienced the sense of isolation—even, admittedly, the hang-ups—that had so affected me. However, she had also seen that the collateral damage I had sustained was only getting worse as time went on. I will forever be grateful to her that she agreed to embark on a move.

We looked around at a few other local churches, without any result. Then at the end of the week of the Cole Classic, we met a couple at a fiftieth birthday party. We ended up in the most absorbing discussion about an 'enlarged' view of the Christian faith as well as the need for the Christian community to better care for the sick and suffering. The wife had suffered gestational diabetes and therefore had real insights into the nature of my illness. Her husband turned out to be the minister of an Anglican church fifteen minutes drive from our home.

The depth of our connection with them that night led me to say to Meredith as we left the party, 'I reckon this night has been an absolute gift—I'd really like to give their church a go.'

We turned up the next Sunday and immediately for me there was no looking back. I felt I had found a Christian community that was putting into action many of the things I had learnt through the wilderness. A real sense of love and community undergirded the gathering. Graciousness exuded from so many of the people there. Here was the kind of church I had longed for—one that felt free to combine the theological and biblical rigour that had so sustained my life with the love, compassion and good works that lay at the heart of the Christian life. Good heads and good hearts. For the first time in about four years, I could breathe clean air again in this area of my life.

More than anything else, this change was a fresh start for me. After the struggle of my illness, the subsequent struggle to find where I fitted in again had gone on for far too long. At our new church, I felt I could begin with a clean slate—no baggage of misunderstanding about my illness, no judgments, no expectations. At last I felt I was accepted just for myself, not on the basis of how useful (or useless) I was.

I had now been on my road back for over three years and I was about to make an important discovery. I was not alone in the struggle to find where to fit in again.

Someone gave me an insightful book that detailed the battle

experience in processing the dislocation brought about
or long-term illness—even after it is thought to be
this book, *Surviving Survival*, was written by a group of
Sydney doctors who had done pioneering work with survivors
of cancer. It identified the very real difficulties involved in reconnecting with life as a survivor.

Their findings resonated deeply with my own experiences. They
reported that 'people registered profound and serious disturbances
in many aspects of their lives'.

*Their sense of identity had been disrupted. It is difficult to exist
as a survivor, because their views and values have changed, while
people around them have not. Their experiences have been such
that they have been made incorrigibly aware of the limitations
and frailties of the human body. The illness had changed the
person they were before the illness.*

They described Edward, a cancer survivor:

*He felt a difference between himself and others, because they
had not confronted human frailty as he had, and they could
not understand the importance of the experience. He could not
communicate its depth. They did not seem to want to enter the
experience with him.*

Towards the end the authors reached this compelling conclusion:

*The first and most common way of handling all this seems to be
the use of 'anchor points', strong values and beliefs that stand
their stead against turbulence.*

This had been exactly my experience. My 'anchor point' was my
knowledge of God, which enabled me to know that there was a big

picture operating way beyond the difficulties and disappointmen of each day. When everything seemed out of control, I was assured of his control. In the middle of loneliness and abandonment, I felt I was never alone. Most importantly, my Christian faith assured me always that there was hope—not just beyond each day's challenges, but hope into eternity.

I can also say with certainty that I could still write about this great hope with assurance and optimism even if I had not 'turned the corner'. Indeed, as I reflect on my years of good health compared with the years of sickness, I think in some ways the life of suffering and vulnerability more accurately represents real life.

In the rush and crush of each day, we imagine that we will last forever. Thanks to remarkable advances in science and medicine, we come to believe our default position is one of health, strength and longevity. But while medical miracles are daily occurrences, we do not last forever. Our days are numbered, as the ancient Hebrew poet wrote so clearly:

> *The length of our days is seventy years—*
> *or eighty, if we have the strength;*
> *yet their span is but trouble and sorrow,*
> *for they quickly pass, and we fly away.*
> *Psalm 90:10–11*

It's not meant to sound morbid—it's the reality of life. Indeed, in my job reporting the upheavals and crises of daily news, I constantly see people deeply shocked to realise that their days so 'quickly pass'.

More than anything else, the experience of chronic fatigue syndrome has allowed me to be more realistic about my very human existence. I have looked deeper into the human condition and learnt rich lessons. We human beings are wonderfully made and remarkably sustained, but we are not invincible. Long-term chronic illness has given me a welcome and crystal clear view of that reality.

Surviving Survival shows that most people who suffer chronic illness come to this kind of realisation. How they respond differs from person to person. For me, it has led to what I see as a much more realistic dependence, not on myself, but on the God who created the universe and who sustains me every day.

Coming to grips with the limitations of the human condition can be a tough challenge. Our human pride makes it difficult for us to admit our boundaries and acknowledge that we are not in control of our destiny. This is why long-term illness can actually turn out to be a blessing. It is something that so strips away our pride and notions of self-sufficiency that we get an entirely new and more realistic view of the temporary nature of our lives.

CFS has forced me to look beyond this frail existence to the sure hope I am promised by the One in whom I trust absolutely. This hope is truly a treasure found in the darkness.

Perhaps for me there was no better way of learning this than with the baffling, infuriating and humbling experience of chronic fatigue syndrome. It remains such an elusive mystery. All I can say from the depths of my being is that, in the midst of much suffering and vulnerability over a long time, God was always there, comforting, reassuring and merciful, always at the right time. Thanks to this, even as my physical suffering deepened, I remained confident, even optimistic, about where it was all leading.

This was not a 'Pollyanna' view or a head-in-the-sand denial of my circumstances. I truly believe it was God assuring me that whatever was going on, it was somehow good for me, even though it hurt—a lot. It was a profound knowledge that things were OK, even if they weren't OK. This didn't happen because I deserved it or had worked for it. It was pure grace—a totally undeserved gift. My fall was indeed a 'fall with grace'.

Those of us who understand the harsh reality of CFS long for the day when it will be more accepted by the medical profession as well as by those around us. Some time after turning the corner, I enthusiastically accepted an invitation to be a patron of the New South Wales Chronic Fatigue Syndrome Society. I have heard our chief patron, the New South Wales governor, Professor Marie Bashir, speak of her earnest desire to see acceptance of the illness, especially within the medical community.

As a psychiatrist, she compares the misunderstandings of CFS to those that used to surround schizophrenia. When she wrote her doctoral thesis in the mid-1960s, it was thought that schizophrenia was caused by the way mothers related to their young babies. Medical science has blown away this dangerous myth, and Professor Bashir says she yearns for the day when the myth that CFS is 'all in the mind' will similarly be blown away.

If CFS remains a challenging illness for those in its grip, it is also extremely challenging for those around the sufferer. This is where I have to pay a monumental tribute to my long-suffering family. For all they have put up with and sacrificed, especially Meredith, I will be forever in their debt. I am also indebted to those wonderful friends who have supported us through my journey.

Regarding those who have been the source of hurt and misunderstanding, much has been forgiven and resolved from my years in the wilderness. Without doubt there is more work to be done, but one of the most attractive things about the Christian life is that it allows the potential for forgiveness. Forgiveness gives me the ability to move on and be free from a consuming bitterness.

It is difficult to know where to rule off a story that in many ways remains a work in progress. For me, in a very real sense, the journey goes on. I am still not back to the health I once knew and am resigned to that and readily accept it.

I have learnt to appreciate my health for the first time, and I work hard to manage the new state of my body. If there is any 'key' to dealing with CFS, in or out of the pit, it is management—knowing your limits and especially respecting them. I now lead a busy, demanding and fulfilling life. Anyone looking at my life could never tell there was anything different about the state of my health. Even so, every so often I have to draw a line in the sand.

As I write in early 2005, we are still as a family sorting through the consequences of this great upheaval in our lives—changed roles, disrupted relationships and unresolved hurts. It is now five years since I 'turned the corner'. For me, it's a vastly improved life for which I will always be grateful. However, you just don't immediately pick up where you left off—either as an individual or as a family. It has been surprising how long and difficult the process has been and may continue to be.

I still struggle to understand it all. Some two years after turning the corner, I went back to see my specialist, Dr Robert Loblay, to report the remarkable turnaround in my health. In the light of everything that had happened, I asked, was it truly chronic fatigue syndrome? He was convinced it was, in all its ill-defined and varied manifestations. 'A multi-headed beast' was the way he described it.

It is very important to say that this book is only my story. My journey out of CFS, using the Glycaemic Index and graded exercise, is *not* the magic key to unlock the mysteries of this illness. Although I have known it to help a number of people, I also know that for very many there is no quick and easy solution. They continue to suffer terribly for years, often for the rest of their lives.

My great desire is that for those still in this wilderness, my story will offer some encouragement, acceptance and hope. Even if their journey goes on and on, my prayer is that they will find ways of knowing: 'It's OK, even if it's not OK.'

APPENDIX

'Meet Me Where I Am'

Caring for those with chronic fatigue or long-term illness

On a Sunday late in the first year of my illness I made one of my increasingly infrequent appearances at church. After the service a friend collared me. 'Your eyes look good,' he said casually. 'Usually when someone is sick you can see it in their eyes.'

His throwaway remark demonstrated two common attitudes of people to my predicament. First, they were genuinely baffled about what was happening to my health. So was I! Many were unrelenting in trying to come up with an explanation and a solution that would see me well again. Second, they seemed to make continual suggestions that my illness was a mental problem, a cop out or a fraud. What else could I make of my friend's comment other than to assume that he didn't really think I was sick at all?

I found all this deeply offensive and tremendously alienating.

Whenever I meet other CFS sufferers, I find they have similar stories to tell. As I have spoken to many who are forced to live with this terrible illness, it is very clear that all the doubts, suspicions and resulting hurt have themselves built a 'community of suffering' entirely independent of the illness itself. All of these people have said this is by far the worst part of the whole experience, notwithstanding considerable physical pain and the loss of normal life.

To the casual or detached observer of chronic fatigue syndrome, it may seem as if I've gone on a great deal, maybe too much, about all these hurts. This is born, not only from my own experiences, but even more deeply from the almost universal experience of other CFS sufferers. I've wanted to be a voice for them, 'crying out in the wilderness'. Here is just one of a myriad of consistent accounts, taken from a letter written by someone courageously battling CFS:

I have experienced many losses, including financial independence, but I think the greatest loss for me has been relationships. Unfortunately, the harshest judgment has come from my immediate family, including my parents . . . because in their eyes I'm just suffering the consequences of my bad choices. It is a bitter grief indeed. I remember lying in bed and thinking, 'I must have some other value than what I can do for God.' My life before getting sick was fun, fulfilling and I believe worthwhile in terms of 'ministry'. I never imagined that there would be anything better. But there is. It is to be loved and valued without being 'useful'.

From my experience, I readily acknowledge that most of those who sought to relate to my family and me were driven by a good heart to help. We can probably also say that generally those who look on and observe long-term illness are driven by an earnest desire to see the suffering brought to an end. The trouble comes when they rush to judgment or ill-informed speculation that makes it sound as if the ill person is somehow responsible for their own predicament.

I think that underneath many of the misjudgments of my own case was the mystery of what was happening to me. People clearly could not handle seeing someone who had been so useful and full of life relegated to being ill for such a long time—and therefore so useless. Equally, people often showed a simple inability to 'meet me where I was'. In the depth of this dreadful illness, the greatest gift that can be offered a sufferer is simple acceptance.

My journals graphically record the darkness of my time in the wilderness. They do not make easy reading. But the process of laboriously wading through them to write this book has shed fresh light for me on both the reality of the illness and my unwavering hope to be well again. It has also fired in me a determination to confront some of the misunderstandings and misjudgments that chronic fatigue sufferers must endure from families, friends and the medical profession.

It is never a comfortable process to rake over other people's mistakes. It is frequently painful. However, in the context of this book, it is important for two reasons. First, to assure those with chronic fatigue syndrome that they are not alone as they suffer both the illness and the destructive attitudes of others. Second, to help those who are alongside sufferers to better know how to react—what to say and do. And more importantly, what not to say and do.

The mistaken notion that CFS is 'all in the mind' or is a choice that the sufferer has made must be exploded. Hopefully my experiences can help do that—as well as suggest a vastly more positive approach that will help rather than harm those suffering chronic fatigue.

Although my condition was a great mystery to me, not everyone seemed to share my puzzlement. A number of visitors repeatedly came with their minds clearly made up about what was 'really' going on in my life.

There were continual oblique references to depression. One of the few work colleagues who kept in touch stopped by and wondered aloud if it was all 'a state of mind'. The very next day, someone spoke to Meredith about 'the mind factor' in my illness.

Another visitor clearly thought I needed to be cheered up and distracted. I found the approach profoundly insulting.

All the time these musings were accompanied by suggestions that if only I could cheer up, psych myself out of it or 'think pleasant thoughts', I would be better again. Those who are in a position to support people with chronic fatigue need to understand how this kind of approach fills them with dismay.

Another deeply distressing thing for sufferers is when people use labels like 'psychological', 'mental' or 'emotional' to describe what is happening in their bodies. In my case, the absence of a specific diagnosis left the field wide open for people to indulge their wildest and most uninformed conjectures. Those who are alongside CFS sufferers at whatever level need to know the harm that careless and unthinking speculation can cause. Drawing their own conclusions in the absence of a clear diagnosis or measurable evidence can be devastating.

Worse still is doubting the reality of this significant and organic illness once the diagnosis is made. And some of the greatest injury comes when the sufferer of CFS (or indeed any illness) is left feeling they have the power to get over it by themselves. This leads to an inevitable conclusion: if the person has the power to fix themselves but is not getting better, they must want to be ill.

Equally damaging is the suggestion that underlying the illness is an aversion to work or life. I sustained a great deal of damage from the constant undercurrent that some people thought I was a bludger or malingerer. These doubts often came through in subtle ways. Several months into my illness, I photocopied some information on ancient Greek for a church minister. When he rang to respond, he began by commenting light-heartedly, 'I think you've clearly got too much time on your hands—I reckon you might be ripping Channel Seven off.' The funny side of this completely escaped me. I found it shockingly insensitive. Much later, when I explained how hurtful the comment had been, he was mortified and apologised profusely.

This episode illustrates how deeply careless words can affect the chronically ill, who perhaps are already, rightly or wrongly, feeling somewhat 'under siege'. Sometimes the words are simply foolish—like the time a friend, growing a beard, told one of my daughters, 'We'll have to get your dad to grow one too to make him feel better.' At other times they are more alarming.

Careless words can significantly increase people's suffering. I vividly recall, for example, something that happened when we were finally able to hook into the income replacement scheme connected with my superannuation insurance. After I explained to someone how the endless paper work often made us feel fraudulent, he replied, 'Yes, and they're probably following you without you knowing it.' When I reported this to Meredith, she said another 'helpful' person had confidently predicted the likelihood that someone would be parked outside our house spying on me.

It is hardly surprising that from then on, in my significantly diminishing world, I developed a bit of paranoia. I had seen plenty of current affairs stories where 'sneaky cam' was used to catch out welfare cheats. This sowed a seed of fear that someone might also concoct a similar story about me. Sometimes I even felt wary of venturing out of the house into the backyard in case I might be being watched!

People need to realise that their words, even those spoken in a throwaway line, can have significant consequences—even if these consequences are sometimes not very rational!

It is important to say that all of this did not mean I was a person who could not be helped. A handful of very special people walked alongside my family and me every step of the journey. They were there, often with impeccable timing, to give us support, both practical and emotional.

They wrote, rang and visited (always checking first if a visit was appropriate). Sometimes they even cooked and gardened for us, helped us out financially, or organised transport for our kids. One dear woman from our church organised for a meal to be dropped around for us every week. Two other families generously offered us the use of holiday apartments, both at the beach. Each offer came at exactly the right time for our family, especially our marriage. For me, a trip to the coast meant a break from the limited confines of home. Just for a while, we breathed some clear air—even sea air!

We were deeply moved by such kindness. People like this were golden. Not surprisingly, we have since become riveted onto some of these new friendships forged in the midst of hardship.

Through all these experiences, both negative and positive, I have learnt a fundamental and critical principle in dealing with those who are ill over the long haul. I call it 'meeting them where they are'. When we are able to leave our opinions, expectations, even our own experiences aside and truly meet those in need where they are, it is a great gift of love, compassion and acceptance.

A piece of wisdom I heard on a taped talk during my illness says it all: 'Most people don't want their problem solved, they want it understood.'

All of the people whom I found supportive and strengthening had grasped this principle. They steadfastly resisted the temptation to rush to judgment, speculation or easy answers. The thing that distinguished them most was that they 'met me where I was'. Although my illness was a mystery to all of us, their concern was to be alongside me and my family in the circumstances of the day and leave the future to God.

They accepted me. They trusted me. They listened—much, much more than they spoke. This was what I needed most.

Out of this came something else indescribably precious. Over and over again, these people would tell me how good it was to be alongside someone walking through the wilderness, gaining insights that were unattainable in the rush and crush of busy lives. In no way is this cause for self-congratulation on my part—purely an indication that the healthy too can benefit if they are able to engage well with those who are doing it tough.

Practically speaking, then, what is helpful and what is not for people going through long-term chronic illness? Sadly, there is no easy answer. One person may draw great strength from a happy, cheery visitor taking their mind off their suffering while another might find such an approach insulting and insufferable.

People sometimes tell me, 'I don't know what to say to someone who's sick.' My reply is, 'You may not need to say much. Your simple presence, especially over the long haul, speaks volumes.' A listening ear amid the urgency and intolerance of modern life is a rare gift. Again, people often ask me, 'What can I do?' My reply is, 'Rather than doing something, sometimes it is much more important just to be there.'

Readily acknowledging that I am not an expert, only someone who has picked up a few insights from being 'in the pit', I offer twelve simple suggestions about how we might better look after those doing it tough.

1. We must recognise that the work of looking after those in need and caring for each other is time-consuming. Quick and self-gratifying solutions are not always the answer.

2. We need to meet people where they are. We may not understand where they are, or why they are there. But they are still entitled to love, respect, care and acceptance.

3. Simple practical help is of immeasurable value. You can never underestimate the power of this—a meal prepared, a garden weeded, the marvellous offer of kids' transport.

4. Letters will often mean much more than a visit or even a call. Hard copy is preferable to emails. Yes, they are hard to write and time-consuming. But over and over again I was lifted up, encouraged and taught, often in exquisitely timed ways, by letters that people had kindly taken the time to pen.

5. For those in the Christian community, prayer is always to be highly valued and, I have no doubt, effective. It is even better if the sick person knows the depth and extent to which people are praying.

6. In my view it is common courtesy and often a necessary kindness for a visitor to ring to see if a visit is appropriate.

7. Remember the spouse and families of the sick person. Often, they are also going through a very tough time. It is good to ask them how they are doing, instead of always inquiring after the person who is ill.

8. Try to resist the understandable temptation to ask 'why?'—and avoid even more trying to come up with answers. Over and over again, I have heard sick people express the simple desire for a willing and understanding ear.

9. Don't speculate. If you don't know what is going on with a person in the midst of illness—for instance, if a diagnosis or prognosis is not clear—resist completely the temptation to come up with your own explanations. And if you do, keep them to yourself entirely. Don't tell the sick person, and definitely don't tell others.

10. Resist anything that might be construed as blaming the sick person for their illness, or for the length of it. This is an easy

trap to fall into and a common problem for many sick people to whom I have spoken.

11. Have an openness to the deep, rich and authentic ways in which the sick, as they move through the wilderness, can be great teachers of the healthy. They are frequently far more in touch with the reality of our human frailty and, if appropriate, a dependence on God.

12. We need to be constantly humble and gracious in how we view this work. I believe we all need to recognise the reality that all of us, at the end of the day, have feet of clay. This even includes those who are sick and prone to rush to judgments, even paranoias, of their own—me included.

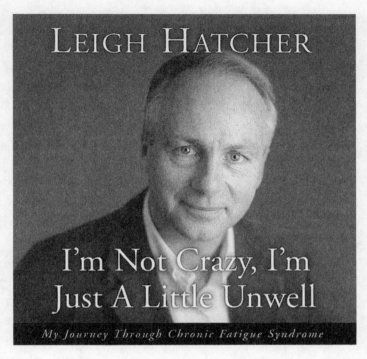

LEIGH HATCHER

I'm Not Crazy, I'm Just A Little Unwell

My Journey Through Chronic Fatigue Syndrome

Many Chronic Fatigue Syndrome sufferers will find the challenge of reading a book very great indeed. 'Brain fog' is a common and debilitating symptom of CFS.

So *I'm Not Crazy, I'm Just a Little Unwell* is also available in a 'talking book'. Hear Leigh Hatcher tell his own story in a CD version of the book or on a downloadable MP3 file. Go to www.notcrazy.net for further details.